RENAL DIET
COOKBOOK

*Healthy Ways To Stop Kidney Disease And
Avoid Dialysis Regardless Of The Stage With Kidney-Friendly
Recipes Low On Potassium, Phosphorus And Sodium*

By
Kristine Peterson

Table Of Contents

Introduction

Chronic kidney disease (CKD) cannot be cured as damages to parts of our kidneys are usually irreversible. However, the good news is that you can slow down the progression of the disease into critical stages by embracing a new lifestyle and way of eating. The kind of foods we eat indubitably has a great effect on the health of our body organs, including the kidneys. As a chronic kidney disease patient, the best thing to do is to switch to a kidney-friendly diet. This kind of diet is popularly known as the renal diet. Although chronic kidney disease cannot be cured, the renal diet can help chronic kidney disease (CKD) patients to retain kidney functions and delay kidney failure for years.

The major effect of the renal diet on our kidneys is that it reduces the workload of the kidney, thereby making them last longer.

A proper renal diet is geared towards reducing the amount of sodium, phosphorus, potassium, protein, and fluid consumed by chronic kidney disease (CKD) patients. When this is achieved, the level of waste released into the blood after the body has extracted the useful materials in the food we eat will reduce. Consequently, the kidney will be relieved as they now have fewer waste products to filter. It would not cost the glomerulus much stress to filter the blood when the level of waste in the blood is low. Human health hangs in a complete balance when all of its interconnected bodily mechanisms function properly in perfect sync. Without its major organs working normally, the body soon suffers permanent damage. Kidney malfunction is one such example, and it is not just the entire water balance that is disturbed by the kidney disease, but a number of other diseases also emerge due to this problem. Kidney diseases are progressive in nature, meaning that if left unchecked and uncontrolled, they can ultimately lead to permanent kidney damage. That is why it is essential to control and manage the disease and put a halt to its progress, which can be done through medicinal and natural means.

While medicines can guarantee only thirty percent of the cure, a change of lifestyle and diet can prove to be miraculous with seventy percent of guaranteed results. A kidney-friendly diet and lifestyle not only saves the kidneys from excess minerals but also aids medicines to work actively. Treatment without a good diet, hence, proves to be useless. In this renal diet cookbook, we shall bring out the basic facts about kidney diseases, their symptoms, causes, and diagnosis. This preliminary introduction can help the readers understand the problem clearly; then, we shall discuss the role of renal diet and kidney-friendly lifestyle in curbing the diseases. And it's not just that. The book also contains a range of delicious renal diet recipes that will guarantee luscious flavors and good health. These include:

- Filtering excess fluids and waste from the blood
- Creating the enzyme known as renin, which regulates blood pressure,
- Ensuring bone marrow creates red blood cells,
- They are controlling calcium and phosphorus levels through absorption and excretion.

Unfortunately, when kidney disease reaches a chronic stage, these functions start to stop working. However, with the right treatment and lifestyle, it is possible to manage symptoms and continue living well. This is even more applicable in the earlier stages of the disease. Tactlessly, 10% of all adults over the age of 20 will experience some form of kidney disease in their lifetime. There are a variety of different treatments for kidney disease, which depend on the cause of the disease. Kidney (or renal) diseases are affecting around 14% of the adult population, according to international stats. In the US, approx. 661.000 Americans suffer from kidney dysfunction. Out of these patients, 468.000 proceed to dialysis treatment, and the rest have one active kidney transplant.

The high quantities of diabetes and heart illness are additionally related to kidney dysfunction, and sometimes one condition, for example, diabetes, may prompt the other. With such a significant number of high rates, possibly the best course of treatment is the contravention of dialysis, which makes people depend upon clinical and crisis facility meds on any occasion multiple times every week.

CHAPTER 1:

Understanding Kidney Disease

Kidney disease is becoming more prevalent in the United States, and so we need to learn as much about it as we can. The more we educate ourselves, the more we can do to take care of this important bodily system. If you've been diagnosed with chronic kidney disease (CKD), education can empower you to most effectively and purposefully manage the disease. Once you have a full understanding of what chronic kidney disease is, you can begin to take charge of your evolving health needs. Making healthy changes early in the stages of kidney disease will help determine how well you will manage your kidney health. I am here to guide you every step of the way. Like any new process, it may seem intimidating at first. But this chapter provides the foundation for learning, and will help you understand kidney disease as you begin your journey to healthier kidneys.

What Do the Kidneys Do?

Our kidneys are small, but they do powerful things to keep our bodies in balance. They are bean-shaped, about the size of a fist, and are located in the middle of the back, on the left and right sides of the spine, just below the rib cage. When everything is working properly, the kidneys do many important jobs such as:

- Filter waste materials from the blood
- Remove extra fluid, or water, from the body
- Release hormones that help manage blood pressure
- Stimulate bone marrow to make red blood cells
- Make an active form of vitamin D that promotes strong, healthy bones

What Causes Kidney Disease?

There are many causes of kidney disease, including physical injury or disorders that can damage the kidneys, but the two leading causes of kidney disease are diabetes and high blood pressure. These underlying conditions also put people at risk for developing cardiovascular disease. Early treatment may not only slow down the progression of the disease but also reduce your risk of developing heart disease or stroke.

Kidney disease can affect anyone at any age. African Americans, Hispanics, and American Indians are at increased risk for kidney failure, because these groups have a greater prevalence of diabetes and high blood pressure.

When we digest protein, our bodies create waste products. As blood flows through the capillaries, the waste products are filtered through the urine. Substances such as protein and red blood cells are too big to pass through the capillaries and so stay in the blood. All the extra work takes a toll on the kidneys. When kidney disease is detected in the early stages, several treatments may prevent the worsening of the disease. If kidney disease is detected in the later stages, high amounts of protein in your urine, called macroalbuminuria, can lead to end-stage renal disease.

The second leading cause of kidney disease is high blood pressure, also known as hypertension. One in three Americans is at risk for kidney disease because of hypertension. Although there is no cure for hypertension, certain medications, a low-sodium diet, and physical activity can lower blood pressure.

The kidneys help manage blood pressure, but when blood pressure is high, the heart has to work overtime at pumping blood. When the force of blood flow is high, blood vessels start to stretch so the blood can flow more easily. The stretching and scarring weaken the blood vessels throughout the entire body, including the kidneys. And when the kidneys' blood vessels are injured, they may not remove the waste and extra fluid from the body, creating a dangerous cycle, because the extra fluid in the blood vessels can increase blood pressure even more.

With diabetes, excess blood sugar remains in the bloodstream. The high blood sugar levels can damage the blood vessels in the kidneys and elsewhere in the body. And since high blood pressure is a complication from diabetes, the extra pressure can weaken the walls of the blood vessels, which can lead to a heart attack or stroke.

Other conditions, such as drug abuse and certain autoimmune diseases, can also cause injury to the kidneys. In fact, every drug we put into our body has to pass through the kidneys for filtration.

An autoimmune disease is one in which the immune system, designed to protect the body from illness, sees the body as an invader and attacks its own systems, including the kidneys. Some forms of lupus, for example, attack the kidneys. Another autoimmune disease that can lead to kidney failure is Good pasture syndrome, a group of conditions that affect the kidneys and the lungs. The damage to the kidneys from autoimmune diseases can lead to chronic kidney disease and kidney failure.

Treatment Plans for Chronic Kidney Disease (CKD)

The best way to manage CKD is to be an active participant in your treatment program, regardless of your stage of renal disease. Proper treatment involves a combination of working with a healthcare team, adhering to a renal diet, and making healthy lifestyle decisions. These can all have a profoundly positive effect on your kidney disease—especially watching how you eat.

Working with your healthcare team. When you have kidney disease, working in partnership with your healthcare team can be extremely important in your treatment program as well as being personally empowering. Regularly meeting with your physician or healthcare team can arm you with resources and information that help you make informed decisions regarding your treatment needs and provides you with a much-needed opportunity to vent, share information, get advice, and receive support in effectively managing this illness.

Adhering to a renal diet. The heart of this book is the renal diet. Sticking to this diet can make a huge difference in your health and vitality. Like any change, following the diet may not be easy at first. Important changes to your diet, particularly early on, can possibly prevent the need for dialysis. These changes include limiting salt, eating a low-protein diet, reducing fat intake, and getting enough calories if you need to lose weight. Be honest with yourself first and foremost—learn what you need, and consider your personal goals and obstacles. Start by making small changes. It is okay to have some slip-ups—we all do. With guidance and support, these small changes will become habits of your promising new lifestyle. In no time, you will begin taking control of your diet and health.

Making healthy lifestyle decisions. Lifestyle choices play a crucial part in our health, especially when it comes to helping regulate kidney disease. Lifestyle choices such as allotting time for physical activity, getting enough sleep, managing weight, reducing stress, and limiting smoking and alcohol will help you take control of your overall health, making it easier to manage your kidney disease. Follow this simple formula: Keep toxins out of your body as much as you can, and build up your immune system with a good balance of exercise, relaxation, and sleep.

CHAPTER 2:

Benefits of Renal Diet

If you have been diagnosed with kidney dysfunction, a proper diet is necessary for controlling the amount of toxic waste in the bloodstream. When toxic waste piles up in the system along with increased fluid, chronic inflammation occurs and we have a much higher chance of developing cardiovascular, bone, metabolic or other health issues.

Since your kidneys can't fully get rid of the waste on their own, which comes from food and drinks, probably the only natural way to help our system is through this diet.

A renal diet is especially useful during the first stages of kidney dysfunction and leads to the following benefits:

Prevents excess fluid and waste build-up

Prevents the progression of renal dysfunction stages

Decreases the likelihood of developing other chronic health problems e.g. heart disorders

Has a mild antioxidant function in the body, which keeps inflammation and inflammatory responses under control.

The above-mentioned benefits are noticeable once the patient follows the diet for at least a month and then continuing it for longer periods, to avoid the stage where dialysis is needed. The strictness of the diet depends on the current stage of renal/kidney disease; if, for example, you are in the 3rd or 4th stage, you should follow a stricter diet and be attentive to the food, which is allowed or prohibited.

These exact foods and nutrients that you should take when following a renal diet, will be given to you in the following sections, and so keep on reading.

Explanation of key diet words

The following nutrients play a major role in a renal diet as some have the ability to improve the condition while others can make it worse. Essentially, a renal diet is based on low consumption of certain nutrients like potassium and phosphorus simply because it promotes fluid buildup within the system of a kidney patient. Here is a brief explanation of the function of each nutrient and its role in a renal diet:

Potassium.

Potassium is a mineral that naturally occurs in certain foods and plays a role in regulating heart rhythm and muscle movement. It is also needed for keeping fluid and electrolyte balance at normal levels. Our kidneys keep only the right levels of potassium in our system, and when it is excess, they expel it via the urine.

The problem is, once kidneys can't function properly, all this excess potassium can't be expelled out and spikes up, causing symptoms like muscle and bone weakness, abnormal heartbeat, and heart failure in extreme cases.

Thus, a diet low in potassium is recommended to prevent buildup and avoid such negative side effects.

Sodium.

Sodium is a trace mineral that is found in most foods that we eat today and it is the key component of salt, which is actually a sodium compound mixed with chloride. Most food that we consume and specially processed food is highly loaded with salt; however, we may be eating sodium in other forms too e.g. fish. The key role of sodium is to regulate blood pressure, help regulate nerve function, and maintain the balance of acids in the blood.

However, when sodium is excessively high and the kidneys can expel it, it can lead to the following symptoms: an elevated feeling of thirst, swelling of hands, feet and the face, elevated blood pressure, and problems with breathing.

This is why it is suggested to keep sodium intake low, to avoid the above.

Phosphorus.

Phosphorus is an essential mineral that is responsible for the development and regeneration of our bones. Phosphorus also plays a key role in the growth of connective tissue e.g. muscles and the regulation of muscle motions. When the food we take contains phosphorus, it gets absorbed by the intestines and then gets deposited in our bones.

However, when kidneys are damaged or dysfunctioning, the excess phosphorus can't be expelled through our systems and causes problems such as: extracting calcium out of the bones/making them weaker, and leading to excess calcium in the bloodstream which interferes with blood vessels, heart, eye, and lung function.

Protein.

Protein is a nutritional compound that consists of amino acids, which play a key role in various system functions like cell communication, oxygen supply, and cellular metabolism. They are also a part of a healthy immune system.

Normally, protein is not an issue for our kidneys. When protein is metabolized, waste by-products are also created and are filtered through the kidneys. This waste along with extrarenal proteins after will be expelled through urine.

However, when kidneys are unable to filter out excess protein, it gets accumulated in the blood and cause problems.

This doesn't mean that renal disease patients should avoid protein totally as it is still necessary for some metabolic functions, as long as it's taken in moderate amounts and based on the stage of renal disease.

Carbs.

Carbs act as a key source of fuel for our bodies. The consumption of carbs is turned into glucose in our system, which is a primary source of energy.

Carbs are ok to be eaten in moderation by kidney patients and the daily recommended allowance is up to 150 grams/day. However, patients that also suffer from Diabetes (besides renal disease) should control their carb consumption to avoid any sudden spikes in their blood glucose.

Fats.

Being in balanced amounts, fats in our bodies act as an energy source, aid in the release of hormones, and help regulate blood pressure.

They also carry some vitamins that are fat-soluble such as A, D, E, and K, which are also very important for our systems. Not all fats are created equal though, some are good for our health and some are bad. Bad fats are saturated and Trans fats and are found in processed meat, dairy, and other products.

They are also found in margarine and vegetable fat shortenings.

Fats, in general, don't pose a risk for renal disease patients; however, it is suggested to limit the consumption of saturated and Tran's fats to avoid any cardiovascular problems e.g. elevated blood pressure and clogging of the arteries.

Dietary fiber.

Dietary fiber is a compound that can't be digested on its own by enzymes and acids in our stomach and intestines, but is needed for the system to aid in the digestion of our food and encourage bowel movements. They generally promote bowel regularity and decrease the likelihood of developing constipation inside the colon. Dietary fiber is typically found in fruits, vegetables, seeds and whole grains.

In patients with renal disease, dietary fiber is ok up to 28 grams/day as long as these plant foods don't contain high amounts of phosphorus or potassium.

Vitamins.

According to medical and dietary guidelines, our bodies need close to 13 vitamins to functions. Vitamins play a key role in metabolic functions and the normal functioning of our cardiovascular, digestive, nervous system and immune systems. The adoption of a nutritionally dense and balanced diet is necessary for getting all the vitamins our system needs. However, due to some diet restrictions e.g. sodium, many renal patients are in need of water-soluble vitamins like B-complex (B1, B2, B6, B12, folic acid, biotin) and small amounts of Vitamin C.

Minerals.

Minerals are needed for our system to maintain healthy connective tissue e.g. bones, muscles, and skin, and facilitate the normal function of our hearts and central nervous systems.

Our kidneys typically expel any excess amount of minerals through our urine as some can lead to health symptoms e.g. muscle spasms when their levels are abnormally high.

However, as it was mentioned earlier, some minerals like potassium and phosphorus cannot be expelled by our kidneys when in excess and so their intake through diet should be limited.

Other trace minerals are perfectly fine when following a renal diet: iron, copper, zinc and selenium. A lack of these can lead to increased oxidative stress and thus, it is important to take sufficient amounts through diet or supplementation.

Fluids.

Fluids are necessary for the proper hydration of our systems in fact; lack of fluids can lead to dehydration and death in extreme cases.

However, in patients with renal dysfunction, fluids can quickly build-up to the point of placing pressure on vital organs like the lungs and heart and becoming dangerous. This is the reason why many physicians advise their kidney patients to limit the consumption of fluids, especially during the last stages of the disorder.

Managing Kidney Disease through Diet

Patients who struggle with kidney health issues, going through kidney dialysis and have renal impairments need to not only go through medical treatment but also change their eating habits, lifestyle to make the situation better. Research has been done on this, and the conclusion is food has a lot to do with how your kidney functions and its overall health.

The first thing to changing your lifestyle is knowing about how your kidney functions and how different food can trigger different reactions in the kidney function. There are certain nutrients that affect your kidney directly. Nutrients like sodium, protein, phosphate, and potassium are the risky ones. You do not have to omit them altogether from your diet, but you need to limit or minimize their intake as much as possible. You cannot leave out essential nutrients like protein from your diet, but you need to count how much protein you are having per day. This is essential in order to keep balance in your muscles and maintaining a good functioning kidney.

A profound change in kidney patients is measuring how much fluid they are drinking. This is a crucial change in every kidney patient, and you must adapt to this new eating habit. Too much water or any other form of liquid can disrupt your kidney function. How much fluid you can consume depends on the condition of your kidney. Most people assign separate bottles for them so that they can measure how much they have drunk and how much more they can drink throughout the day.

CHAPTER 3:

Stages of Kidney Disease

According to the National Kidney Foundation in the US, kidney disease can be classified into five different progressive stages. These stages and their symptoms do not only help the doctor to devise an appropriate therapy but also guide the patient to take the necessary measures in routine life. The rate of kidney function actually tells much about these phases. In the early stages, there is minimum loss of function, and this loss increases with every stage.

The eGFR is used as a standard criterion to measure the Kidney function. EGFR is the acronym for the estimated Glomerular Filtration Rate. It is the rate at which the waste material is transferred from the blood to the nephron's tubes through the "glomerulus"- the filtering membrane of the kidney tissues. The lesser the rate of glomerular filtration, the greater the problem the kidneys are going through. A person's age, gender, race, and serum creatinine are entered into a mathematical formula to calculate his eGFR. The serum creatinine level is measured in a blood test. The creatinine is actually a waste product of the body which is produced out of muscular activities. Healthy kidneys are capable of removing all the creatinine out of the blood. A rising creatinine level is therefore a sign of kidney disease. It is said that if a person has been having an eGFR of less than 60 for three months, it means that he is suffering from serious renal problems. The five main stages of chronic kidney disease can be categorized as follows:

- Stage 1:

The first stage starts when the eGFR gets slightly higher than the normal value. In this stage, the eGFR can be equal to or greater than 90mL/min

- Stage 2:

The next stage arises when the eGFR starts to decline and ranges between 60 to 89 mL/min. It is best to control the progression of the disease at this point.

- Stage 3:

From this point on, the kidney disease becomes concerning for the patient as the eGFR drops to 30-59 mL/min. At this stage, consultation is essential for the health of the patient.

- Stage 4:

Stage 4 is also known as Severe Chronic Kidney Disease as the eGFR level drops to 15-29 mL/min.

- Stage 5:

The final and most critical phase of chronic renal disease is stage 5, where the estimated glomerular filtration rate gets as low as below 15 mL/min.

Role of Potassium, Sodium, and Phosphorous

1. Sodium

Sodium is considered the most important electrolyte of the body next to chloride and potassium. The electrolytes are actually the substance that controls the flow of fluids into the cells and out of them. Sodium is mainly responsible for regulating blood volume and pressure. It is also involved in controlling muscle contraction and nerve functions. The acid-base balance in the blood and other body fluids is also regulated by sodium. Though sodium is important for the health and regulation of important body mechanisms, excessive sodium intake, especially when a person suffers from some stages of chronic kidney disease, can be dangerous. Excess sodium disrupts the critical fluid balance in the body and inside the kidneys. It then leads to high blood pressure, which in turn negatively affects the kidneys. Salt is one of the major sources of sodium in our diet, and it is strictly forbidden on the renal diet. High sodium intake can also lead to Edema, which is swelling of the face, hands, and legs. Furthermore, high blood pressure can stress the heart and cause the weakening of its muscles. The build-up of fluid in the lungs also leads to shortness of breath.

2. Potassium

Potassium is another mineral that is closely linked to renal health. Potassium is another important electrolyte, so it maintains the fluid balance in the body and its pH levels as well. This electrolyte also plays an important role in controlling nerve impulses and muscular activity. It works in conjugation with the sodium to carry out all these functions. The normal potassium level in the blood must range between 3.5 and 5.5mEq/L. It is the kidneys that help maintain this balance, but without their proper function, the potassium starts to build up in the blood. Hyperkalemia is a condition characterized by high potassium levels. It usually occurs in people with chronic kidney disease. The prominent symptoms of high potassium are numbness, slow pulse rate, weakness, and nausea. Potassium is present in green vegetables and some fruits, and these ingredients should be avoided on a renal diet.

3. Phosphorous

The amount of phosphorus in the blood is largely linked to the functioning of the kidneys. Phosphorus, in combination with vitamin D, calcium, and parathyroid hormone, can regulate renal function. The balance of phosphorous and calcium is maintained by the kidneys, and this balance keeps the bones and teeth healthy. Phosphorous, along with vitamin D, ensures the absorption of calcium into the bones and teeth, where this mineral is important for the body. On the other hand, it gets dangerous when the kidneys fail to control the amount of phosphorus in the blood. This may lead to heart and bone-related problems. Mainly there is a high risk of weakening of the bones followed by the hardening of the tissues due to the deposition of phosphorous and calcium outside the bones. This abnormal calcification can occur in the lungs, skin, joints, and arteries, which can become in time very painful. It may also result in bone pain and itching.

CHAPTER 4:

What you can Eat, What to Avoid

Foods You Need

There are many foods that work well within the renal diet, and once you see the available variety, it will not seem as restrictive or difficult to follow. The key is focusing on the foods with a high level of nutrients, which make it easier for the kidneys to process waste by not adding too much that the body needs to discard. Balance is a major factor in maintaining and improving long-term renal function.

Garlic

Excellent, vitamin-rich food for the immune system, garlic is a tasty substitute for salt in a variety of dishes. It acts as a significant source of vitamin C and B6 while aiding the kidneys in ridding the body of unwanted toxins. It's a great, healthy way to add flavor to skillet meals, pasta, soups, and stews.

Berries

All berries are considered a good renal diet food due to their high level of fiber, antioxidants, and delicious taste, making them an easy option to include as a light snack or as an ingredient in smoothies, salads, and light desserts. Just one handful of blueberries can provide almost one day's vitamin C requirement, as well as a boost of fiber, which is good for weight loss and maintenance.

Bell Peppers

Flavorful and easy to enjoy both raw and cooked, bell peppers offer a good source of vitamin C, vitamin A, and fiber. Along with other kidney-friendly foods, they make the detoxification process much easier while boosting your body's nutrient level to prevent further health conditions and reduce existing deficiencies.

Onions

This nutritious and tasty vegetable is excellent as a companion to garlic in many dishes, or on its own. Like garlic, onions can provide flavor as an alternative to salt, and provides a good source of vitamin C, vitamin B, manganese, and fiber, as well. Adding just one quarter or half of the onion is often enough for most meals because of its strong, pungent flavor.

Macadamia Nuts

If you enjoy nuts and seeds as snacks, you may soon learn that many contain high amounts of phosphorus and should be avoided or limited as much as possible. Fortunately, macadamia nuts are an easier option to digest and process, as they contain much lower amounts of phosphorus and make an excellent substitute for other nuts. They are a good source of other nutrients, as well, such as vitamin B, copper, manganese, iron, and healthy fats.

Pineapple

Unlike other fruits that are high in potassium, pineapple is an option that can be enjoyed more often than bananas and kiwis. Citrus fruits are generally high in potassium as well, so if you find yourself craving an orange or grapefruit, choose pineapple instead. In addition to providing high levels of vitamin B and fiber, pineapples can reduce inflammation thanks to an enzyme called bromelain.

Mushrooms

In general, mushrooms are a safe, healthy option for the renal diet, especially the shiitake variety, which are high in nutrients such as selenium, vitamin B, and manganese. They contain a moderate amount of plant-based protein, which is easier for your body to digest and use than animal proteins. Shiitake and Portobello mushrooms are often used in vegan diets as a meat substitute due to their texture and pleasant flavor.

Foods you Need to Avoid

Eating restrictions might be different depending upon your level of kidney disease. If you are in the early stages of kidney disease, you may have different restrictions as compared to those who are at the end-stage renal disease or kidney failure. In contrast to this, people with an end-stage renal disease requiring dialysis will face different eating restrictions. Let's discuss some of the foods to avoid while being on the renal diet.

Dark-Colored Colas contain calories, sugar, phosphorus, etc. They contain phosphorus to enhance flavor, increase their life, and avoid discoloration. Which can be found in a product's ingredient list. This addition of phosphorus varies depending on the type of cola. Mostly, the dark-colored colas contain 50–100 mg in a 200-ml serving. Therefore, dark colas should be avoided on a renal diet.

Canned Foods including soups, vegetables, and beans, are low in cost but contain high amounts of sodium due to the addition of salt to increase its life. Due to this amount of sodium inclusion in canned goods, it is better that people with kidney disease should avoid consumption. Opt for lower-sodium content with the label "no salt added". One more way is to drain or rinse canned foods, such as canned beans and tuna, which could decrease the sodium content by 33–80%, depending on the product.

Brown Rice is a whole grain containing a higher concentration of potassium and phosphorus than its white rice counterpart. One cup of already cooked brown rice possesses about 150 mg of phosphorus and 154 mg of potassium, whereas, one cup of already cooked white rice has an amount of about 69 mg of phosphorus and 54 mg of potassium. Bulgur, buckwheat, pearled barley and couscous are equally beneficial, low-phosphorus options and might be a good alternative instead of brown rice.

Bananas are high potassium content, low in sodium, and provides 422 mg of potassium per banana. It might disturb your daily balanced potassium intake to 2,000 mg if a banana is a daily staple.

Whole-Wheat Bread may harm individuals with kidney disease. But for healthy individuals, it is recommended over refined, white flour bread. White bread is recommended instead of whole-wheat varieties for individuals with kidney disease just because it has phosphorus and potassium. If you add more bran and whole grains to the bread, then the amount of phosphorus and potassium contents goes higher.

Oranges and Orange Juice are enriched with vitamin C content and potassium. 184 grams provides 333 mg of potassium and 473 mg of potassium in one cup of orange juice. With these calculations, oranges and orange juice must be avoided or used in a limited amount while being on a renal diet.

Some of the high-potassium foods, likewise potatoes and sweet potatoes, could also be soaked or leached to lessen the concentration of potassium contents. Cut them into small and thin pieces and boil those for at least 10 minutes can reduce the potassium content by about 50%. Potatoes that are soaked in a wide pot of water for as low as four hours before cooking could possess even less potassium content than those not soaked before cooking. This is known as "potassium leaching," or the "double cook Direction."

If you are suffering from or living with kidney disease, reducing your potassium, phosphorus and sodium intake is an essential aspect of managing and tackling the disease. The foods with high-potassium, high-sodium, and high-phosphorus content listed above should always be limited or avoided. These restrictions and nutrients intakes may differ depending on the level of damage to your kidneys. Following a renal diet might be a daunting procedure and a restrictive one most of the time. But, working with your physician and nutrition specialist and a renal dietitian can assist you in formulating a renal diet specific to your individual needs.

Renal Diet Shopping List

Vegetables:

- Arugula (raw)
- Alfalfa sprouts
- Bamboo shoots
- Asparagus
- Beans - pinto, wax, fava, green
- Bean sprouts
- Bitter melon (balsam pear)
- Beet greens (raw)
- Broccoli
- Broad beans (boiled, fresh)

- Cactus
- Cabbage - red, swamp, Napa/ Suey Choy, skunk
- Carrots
- Calabash
- Celery
- Cauliflower
- Chayote
- Celeriac (cooked)
- Collard greens
- Chicory
- Cucumber
- Corn
- Okra
- Onions
- Pepitas
- (Green) Peas
- Peppers
- Radish
- Radicchio
- Seaweed
- Rapini (raw)
- Shallots
- Spinach (raw)
- Snow peas
- Dandelion greens (raw)
- Daikon
- Plant Leaves

- Drumstick
- Endive
- Eggplant
- Fennel bulb
- Escarole
- Fiddlehead greens
- Ferns
- Hearts of Palm
- Irish moss
- Hominy
- Jicama, raw
- Leeks
- Kale(raw)
- Mushrooms (raw white)
- Lettuce (raw)
- Mustard greens
- Swiss chard (raw)
- Squash
- Turnip
- Tomatillos (raw)
- Watercress
- Turnip greens
- Wax beans
- Water chestnuts (canned)
- Winter melon
- Wax gourd
- Zucchini (raw)

Fruits:
- Acerola Cherries
- Apple
- Blackberries
- Asian Pear
- Boysenberries
- Blueberries
- Cherries
- Casaba melon
- Clementine
- Chokeberries
- Crabapples
- Cloudberries
- Cranberries (fresh)
- Grapefruit
- Gooseberries
- Pomegranate
- Grapes
- Rambutan
- Quince

- Rhubarb
- Raspberries (fresh or frozen)
- Jujubes
- Golden Berry
- Kumquat
- Jackfruit
- Lingonberries
- Lemon
- Loganberries
- Lime
- Lychees
- Mango
- Mandarin orange
- Peach
- Pineapple
- Pear
- Plum
- Strawberries
- Rose-apple

- Tangerine
- Tangelo
- Watermelon

Fresh Meat, Seafood, and Poultry:

- Chicken
- Beef and Ground Beef
- Goat
- Duck
- Wild Game
- Pork
- Lamb
- Veal
- Turkey
- Fish

Milk, Eggs, and Dairy:

Milk:

- Milk (½-1 cup/day)

Non-Dairy Milk:

- Almond Fresh (Original, Unsweetened, Vanilla)
- Almond Breeze (Original, Vanilla, Vanilla Unsweetened, Original Unsweetened)
- Silk True Almond Beverage (Unsweetened Original, Original, Vanilla, Unsweetened Vanilla)
- Good Karma Flax Delight (Vanilla, Original, Unsweetened)
- Rice Dream Rice Drink (Vanilla Classic, Non-Enriched Original Classic)
- Silk Soy Beverage (Original, Vanilla, Unsweetened)
- Natura Organic Fortified Rice Beverage (Original, Vanilla)
- PC Organics Fortified Rice Beverage

Other Dairy Products:

- Non-Hydrogenated Margarine (Salt-Free or Regular)
- Butter (Unsalted or Regular)
- Whipping Cream
- Sour Cream
- Whipped Cream

CHAPTER 5:

Breakfast

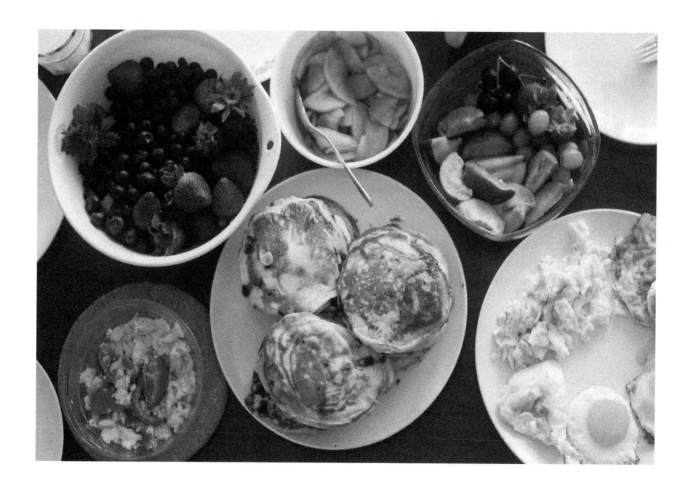

Mozzarella Cheese Omelet

Preparation Time: 10 minutes
Cooking Time: 5 minutes
Servings: 1
Ingredients:

- 4 eggs, beaten
- 1/4 cup mozzarella cheese, shredded
- 4 red pepper slices
- 1/4 tsp. Italian seasoning
- 1/4 tsp. dried oregano
- Pepper
- Salt

Directions:

1. In a small bowl, whisk eggs with salt.
2. Spray pan with cooking spray and heat over medium heat.
3. Pour egg mixture into the pan and cook over medium heat.
4. Once eggs are set then sprinkle oregano and Italian seasoning on top.
5. Arrange red pepper slices on top of the omelet and sprinkle with shredded cheese.
6. Cook omelet for 1 minute. Serve and enjoy.

Nutrition:

Calories 285 Fat 19g Carbs 4g
Protein 25g Phosphorus 22mg Potassium 32mgSodium 12 mg

Sun-Dried Red pepper Frittata

Preparation Time: 10 minutes
Cooking Time: 20 minutes
Servings: 8
Ingredients:

- 12 eggs
- 1/2 tsp. dried basil
- 1/4 cup parmesan cheese, grated
- 2 cups baby spinach, shredded
- 1/4 cup sun-dried red peppers, sliced
- Pepper - Salt

Directions:

1. Preheat the oven to 425 F. In a large bowl, whisk eggs with pepper and salt.
2. Add remaining ingredients and stir to combine. Spray oven-safe pan with cooking spray.

3. Pour egg mixture into the pan and bake for 20 minutes. Slice and serve.

Nutrition:

Calories 115 Fat 7g Carbs 1g Protein 10g Phosphorus 22mg Potassium 32mg Sodium 12 mg

Italian Breakfast Frittata

Preparation Time: 10 minutes
Cooking Time: 45 minutes
Servings: 4
Ingredients:

- 2 cups egg whites
- 1/2 cup mozzarella cheese, shredded
- 1 cup cottage cheese, crumbled
- 1/4 cup fresh basil, sliced
- 1/2 cup roasted red peppers, sliced
- Pepper
- Salt

Directions:

1. Preheat the oven to 375 F.
2. Add all ingredients into the large bowl and whisk well to combine.
3. Pour frittata mixture into the baking dish and bake for 45 minutes.
4. Slice and serve.

Nutrition:

Calories 131 Fat 2g Carbs 5g
Protein 22g Phosphorus: 22mg Potassium 32mgSodium 12mg

Sausage Cheese Bake Omelet

Preparation Time: 10 minutes
Cooking Time: 45 minutes
Servings: 8
Ingredients:

- 16 eggs
- 2 cups cheddar cheese, shredded
- 1/2 cup salsa
- 1 lb. ground sausage
- 1 1/2 cups coconut milk
- Pepper
- Salt

Directions:

1. Preheat the oven to 350 F.
2. Add sausage in a pan and cook until browned. Drain excess fat.
3. In a large bowl, whisk eggs and milk. Stir in cheese, cooked sausage, and salsa.
4. Pour omelet mixture into the baking dish and bake for 45 minutes.
5. Serve and enjoy.

Nutrition:

Calories 360 Fat 24g Carbs 4g
Phosphorus: 22mg Potassium 32mg Sodium 12mg Protein 28g

Greek Egg Scrambled

Preparation Time: 10 minutes
Cooking Time: 10 minutes
Servings: 2
Ingredients:

- 4 eggs
- 1/2 cup grape red peppers, sliced
- 2 tbsp. green onions, sliced
- 1 bell pepper, diced
- 1 tbsp. caper oil
- 1/4 tsp. dried oregano
- 1/2 tbsp. capers
- 3 capers, sliced
- Pepper
- Salt

Directions:

1. Heat oil in a pan over medium heat
2. Add green onions and bell pepper and cook until pepper is softened.
3. Add red peppers, capers, and capers and cook for 1 minute.
4. Add eggs and stir until eggs are cooked. Season it with oregano, pepper, and salt.
5. Serve and enjoy.

Nutrition:

Calories 230 Fat 17g Carbs 8g Phosphorus: 22mg Potassium 32mg Sodium 12 mg Protein 12g

Feta Mint Omelet

Preparation Time: 10 minutes
Cooking Time: 5 minutes
Servings: 1
Ingredients:

- 3 eggs
- 1/4 cup fresh mint, chopped
- 2 tbsp. coconut milk
- 1/2 tsp. caper oil
- 2 tbsp. feta cheese, crumbled
- Pepper
- Salt

Directions:

1. In a bowl, whisk eggs with feta cheese, mint, milk, pepper, and salt.
2. Heat caper oil in a pan over low heat. Pour egg mixture in the pan and cook until eggs are set.
3. Flip omelet and cook for 2 minutes more.
4. Serve and enjoy.

Nutrition:

Calories 275 Fat 20g Phosphorus 22mg Potassium 32mg
Sodium 12 mg Carbs 4g Protein 20g

Sausage Breakfast Casserole

Preparation Time: 10 minutes
Cooking Time: 50 minutes
Servings: 8
Ingredients:

- 12 eggs
- 1 lb. ground Italian sausage
- 2 1/2 red peppers, sliced
- 3 tbsp. coconut flour
- 1/4 cup coconut milk
- 2 small zucchinis, shredded
- Pepper
- Salt

Directions:

1. Preheat the oven to 350 F.
2. Spray casserole dish with cooking spray and set aside.
3. Cook sausage in a pan until brown.
4. Transfer sausage to a mixing bowl.

5. Add coconut flour, milk, eggs, zucchini, pepper, and salt. Stir well.
6. Add eggs and whisk to combine.
7. Transfer bowl mixture into the casserole dish and top with red pepper slices.
8. Bake for 50 minutes.
9. Serve and enjoy.

Nutrition:
Calories 305 Fat 21.8g Carbs 6.3g
Phosphorus 22mg Potassium 32mg Sodium 12 mg Protein 19.6g

Easy Turnip Puree
Preparation Time: 10 minutes
Cooking Time: 12 minutes
Servings: 4
Ingredients:

- 1 1/2 lbs. turnips, peeled and chopped
- 1 tsp. dill
- 3 bacon slices, cooked and chopped
- 2 tbsp. fresh chives, chopped

Directions:

1. Add turnip into the boiling water and cook for 12 minutes. Drain well and place in a food processor.
2. Add dill and process until smooth.
3. Transfer turnip puree into the bowl and top with bacon and chives.
4. Serve and enjoy.

Nutrition:
Calories 127 Fat 6g Carbs 11.6g
Phosphorus: 22mg Potassium 32mg Sodium 12 mg Protein 6.8g

Spinach Bacon Breakfast Bake
Preparation Time: 10 minutes
Cooking Time: 45 minutes
Servings: 6
Ingredients:

- 10 eggs
- 3 cups baby spinach, chopped
- 1 tbsp. caper oil
- 8 bacon slices, cooked and chopped
- 2 red peppers, sliced
- 2 tbsp. chives, chopped
- Pepper - Salt

Directions:

1. Preheat the oven to 350 F.
2. Spray a baking dish with cooking spray and set aside.
3. Heat oil in a pan
4. Add spinach and cook until spinach wilted.
5. In a mixing bowl, whisk eggs and salt. Add spinach and chives and stir well.
6. Pour egg mixture into the baking dish.
7. Top with red peppers and bacon and bake for 45 minutes.
8. Serve and enjoy.

Nutrition:
Calories 273 Fat 20.4g Carbs 3.1g Phosphorus: 12mg
Potassium 32mg Sodium 22mg Protein 19.4g

Healthy Spinach Red Pepper Muffins
Preparation Time: 10 minutes
Cooking Time: 20 minutes
Servings: 12
Ingredients:

- 12 eggs
- 1/2 tsp. Italian seasoning
- 1 cup red peppers, chopped
- 4 tbsp. water
- 1 cup fresh spinach, chopped
- Pepper - Salt

Directions:

1. Preheat the oven to 350 F. Spray a muffin tray with cooking spray and set aside.
2. In a mixing bowl, whisk eggs with water, Italian seasoning, pepper, and salt.
3. Add spinach and red peppers and stir well. Pour egg mixture into the prepared muffin tray and bake for 20 minutes. Serve and enjoy.

Nutrition:
Calories 67 Fat 4.5g Carbs 1g Phosphorus: 12mg
Potassium 32mg Sodium 22 mg Protein 5.7g

Chicken Egg Breakfast Muffins

Preparation Time: 10 minutes
Cooking Time: 15 minutes
Servings: 12
Ingredients:

- 10 eggs
- 1 cup cooked chicken, chopped
- 3 tbsp. green onions, chopped
- 1/4 tsp. garlic powder
- Pepper
- Salt

Directions:

1. Preheat the oven to 400 F.
2. Spray a muffin tray with cooking spray and set aside.
3. In a large bowl, whisk eggs with garlic powder, pepper, and salt.
4. Add remaining ingredients and stir well.
5. Pour egg mixture into the muffin tray and bake for 15 minutes.
6. Serve and enjoy.

Nutrition:
Calories 71 Fat 4 g
Carbs 0.4g Phosphorus 12mg
Potassium 32mgSodium 22mg
Protein 8g

Breakfast Egg Salad

Preparation Time: 10 minutes
Cooking Time: 5 minutes
Servings: 4
Ingredients:

- 6 eggs, hard-boiled, peeled and chopped
- 1 tbsp. fresh dill, chopped
- 4 tbsp. mayonnaise
- Pepper
- Salt

Directions:

1. Add all ingredients into the large bowl and stir to mix. Serve and enjoy.

Nutrition:
Calories 140 Fat 10g
Carbs 4g Protein 8g
Phosphorus: 12mg
Potassium 32mg
Sodium 22mg

Vegetable Tofu Scramble

Preparation Time: 10 minutes
Cooking Time: 7 minutes
Servings: 2
Ingredients:

- 1/2 block firm tofu, crumbled
- 1/4 tsp. ground cumin
- 1 tbsp. turmeric
- 1 cup spinach
- 1/4 cup zucchini, chopped
- 1 tbsp. caper oil
- 1 red pepper, chopped
- 1 tbsp. chives, chopped
- 1 tbsp. coriander, chopped
- Pepper
- Salt

Directions:

2. Heat oil in a pan over medium heat
3. Add red pepper, zucchini, and spinach and sauté for 2 minutes.
4. Add tofu, cumin, turmeric, pepper, and salt and sauté for 5 minutes.
5. Top with chives, and coriander.
6. Serve and enjoy.

Nutrition:
Calories 101
Fat 8.5g
Carbs 5.1g
Phosphorus 12mg
Potassium 32mg
Sodium 22 mg
Protein 3.1g

Cheese Coconut Pancakes

Preparation Time: 10 minutes
Cooking Time: 5 minutes
Servings: 1
Ingredients:

- 2 eggs
- 1 packet stevia
- 1/2 tsp. cinnamon
- 2 oz. cream cheese
- 1 tbsp. coconut flour
- 1/2 tsp. vanilla

Directions:
1. Add all ingredients into the bowl and blend until smooth.
2. Spray pan with cooking spray and heat over medium-high heat.
3. Pour batter on the hot pan and make two pancakes.
4. Cook pancake until lightly brown from both the sides.
5. Serve and enjoy.

Nutrition:
Calories 386 Fat 30g
Phosphorus: 12mg Potassium 32mg
Sodium 22mgCarbs 12g
Sugar 1g Protein 16g

Cheesy Scrambled Eggs with Fresh Herbs

Preparation Time: 15 minutes
Cooking Time: 10 minutes
Servings: 4
Ingredients:

- Eggs – 3
- Egg whites – 2
- Cream cheese – 1/2 cup
- Unsweetened rice milk – 1/4 cup
- Chopped scallion – 1 Tbsp. green part only
- Chopped fresh tarragon – 1 Tbsp.
- Unsalted butter – 2 Tbsps.
- Ground black pepper to taste

Directions:
1. In a bowl, whisk the eggs, egg whites, cream cheese, rice milk, scallions, and tarragon until mixed and smooth.
2. Melt the butter in a skillet.
3. Pour in the egg mixture and cook, stirring, for 5 minutes or until the eggs are thick and curds creamy.
4. Season with pepper and serve.

Nutrition:
Calories 221 Fat 19g
Carbs 3g Phosphorus 119mg
Potassium 140mg Sodium 193mg
Protein 8g

Coconut Breakfast Smoothie

Preparation Time: 5 minutes
Cooking Time: 5 minutes
Servings: 1
Ingredients:

- 1/4 cup whey protein powder
- 1/2 cup coconut milk
- 5 drops liquid stevia
- 1 tbsp. coconut oil
- 1 tsp. vanilla
- 2 tbsp. coconut butter
- 1/4 cup water
- 1/2 cup ice

Directions:
1. Add all ingredients into the blender and blend until smooth.
2. Serve and enjoy.

Nutrition:
Calories 560
Fat 45g
Carbs 12g
Phosphorus: 12mg
Potassium 32mg
Sodium 22 mg
Protein 25g

Turkey and Spinach Scramble on Melba Toast

Preparation Time: 2 minutes
Cooking Time: 15 minutes
Servings: 2
Ingredients:

- Extra virgin caper oil – 1 tsp.
- Raw spinach – 1 cup
- Garlic – 1/2 clove, minced
- Nutmeg – 1 tsp. grated
- Cooked and diced turkey breast – 1 cup
- Melba toast – 4 slices
- Balsamic vinegar – 1 tsp.

Directions:
1. Heat a skillet over medium heat and add oil.
2. Add turkey and heat through for 6 to 8 minutes.

3. Add spinach, garlic, and nutmeg and stir-fry for 6 minutes more.
4. Plate up the Melba toast and top with spinach and turkey scramble.
5. Drizzle with balsamic vinegar and serve.

Nutrition:
Calories 301
Fat 19g
Carbs 12g
Phosphorus 215mg
Potassium 269mg
Sodium 360mg
Protein 19g

Vegetable Omelet

Preparation Time: 15 minutes
Cooking Time: 10 minutes
Servings: 3
Ingredients:

- Egg whites – 4
- Egg – 1
- Chopped fresh parsley – 2 Tbsps.
- Water – 2 Tbsps.
- Caper oil spray
- Chopped and boiled red bell pepper – 1/2 cup
- Chopped scallion – 1/4 cup, both green and white parts
- Ground black pepper

Directions:

1. Whisk together the egg, egg whites, parsley, and water until well blended. Set aside.
2. Spray a skillet with caper oil spray and place over medium heat.
3. Sauté the peppers and scallion for 3 minutes or until softened.
4. Pour the egg mixture into the skillet over vegetables and cook, swirling the skillet, for 2 minutes or until the edges start to set. Cook until set.
5. Season with black pepper and serve.

Nutrition:
Calories 77 Fat 3g Carbs 2g Phosphorus 67mg
Potassium 194mg Sodium 229mg Protein 12g

Mexican Style Burritos

Preparation Time: 5 minutes
Cooking Time: 15 minutes
Servings: 2
Ingredients:

- Caper oil – 1 Tbsp.
- Corn tortillas – 2
- Red onion – 1/4 cup, chopped
- Red bell peppers – 1/4 cup, chopped
- Red chili – 1/2, deseeded and chopped
- Eggs – 2
- Juice of 1 lime
- Cilantro – 1 Tbsp. chopped

Directions:

1. Turn the broiler to medium heat and place the tortillas underneath for 1 to 2 minutes on each side or until lightly toasted.
2. Remove and keep the broiler on.
3. Heat the oil in a skillet and sauté onion, chili and bell peppers for 5 to 6 minutes or until soft.
4. Crack the eggs over the top of the onions and peppers and place skillet under the broiler for 5 to 6 minutes or until the eggs are cooked.
5. Serve half the eggs and vegetables on top of each tortilla and sprinkle with cilantro and lime juice to serve.

Nutrition:
Calories 202 Fat 13g Carbs 19g
Phosphorus 184mg Potassium 233mg
Sodium 77mg Protein 9g

Bulgur, Couscous and Buckwheat Cereal

Preparation Time: 10 minutes
Cooking Time: 25 minutes
Servings: 4
Ingredients:

- Water – 2 1/4 cups
- Vanilla rice milk – 1 1/4 cups
- Uncooked bulgur – 6 Tbsps.

- Uncooked whole buckwheat – 2 Tbsps.
- Sliced apple – 1 cup
- Plain uncooked couscous – 6 Tbsps.
- Ground cinnamon – 1/2 tsp.

Directions:

1. In a saucepan, heat the water and milk over medium heat.
2. Bring to a boil, and add the bulgur, buckwheat, and apple.
3. Reduce the heat to low and simmer, occasionally stirring until the bulgur is tender, about 20 to 25 minutes.
4. Remove the saucepan from the heat and stir in the couscous and cinnamon.
5. Let the saucepan stand, covered, for 10 minutes.
6. Fluff the cereal with a fork before serving.

Nutrition:
Calories 159
Fat 1g
Carbs 34g
Phosphorus 130mg
Potassium 116mg
Sodium 33mg
Protein 4g

Sweet Pancakes

Preparation Time: 10 minutes
Cooking Time: 5 minutes
Servings: 5
Ingredients:

- All-purpose flour – 1 cup
- Granulated sugar – 1 Tbsp.
- Baking powder – 2 tsps.
- Egg whites – 2
- Almond milk - 1 cup
- Caper oil - 2 Tbsps.
- Maple extract – 1 Tbsp.

Directions:

1. Mix the flour, sugar and baking powder in a bowl.
2. Make a well in the center and place to one side.

3. In another bowl, mix the egg whites, milk, oil, and maple extract.
4. Add the egg mixture to the well and gently mix until a batter is formed.
5. Heat skillet over medium heat.
6. Add 1/5 of the batter to the pan and cook 2 minutes on each side or until the pancake is golden.
7. Repeat with the remaining batter and serve.

Nutrition:
Calories 178
Fat 6g
Carbs 25g
Phosphorus 116mg
Potassium 126mg
Sodium 297mg
Protein 6g

Breakfast Smoothie

Preparation Time: 15 minutes
Cooking Time: 0 minutes
Servings: 2
Ingredients:

- Frozen blueberries – 1 cup
- Pineapple chunks – 1/2 cup
- English cucumber – 1/2 cup
- Apple – 1/2
- Water – 1/2 cup

Directions:

1. Put the pineapple, blueberries, cucumber, apple, and water in a blender and blend until thick and smooth.
2. Pour into 2 glasses and serve.

Nutrition:
Calories: 87
Fat 0g
Carbs 22g
Phosphorus: 28mg
Potassium: 192mg
Sodium: 3mg
Protein: 0.7g

Buckwheat and Grapefruit Porridge
Preparation Time: 5 minutes
Cooking Time: 20 minutes
Servings: 2
Ingredients:

- Buckwheat – 1/2 cup
- Grapefruit – 1/4, chopped
- Honey – 1 Tbsp.
- Almond milk – 1 1/2 cups
- Water – 2 cups

Directions:

1. Bring the water to a boil on the stove. Add the buckwheat and place the lid on the pan.
2. Lower heat slightly and simmer for 7 to 10 minutes, checking to ensure water does not dry out.
3. When most of the water is absorbed, remove and set aside for 5 minutes.
4. Drain any excess water from the pan and stir in almond milk, heating through for 5 minutes.
5. Add the honey and grapefruit.
6. Serve.

Nutrition:
Calories 231
Fat 4g
Carbs 43g
Phosphorus 165mg
Sodium 22mg
Potassium 370mg
Sodium 135mg

Egg and Veggie Muffins
Preparation Time: 15 minutes
Cooking Time: 20 minutes
Servings: 4
Ingredients:

- Cooking spray
- Eggs – 4
- Unsweetened rice milk – 2 Tbsp.
- Sweet onion – 1/2, chopped
- Red bell pepper – 1/2, chopped
- Pinch red pepper flakes
- Pinch ground black pepper

Directions:

1. Preheat the oven to 350F.
2. Spray 4 muffin pans with cooking spray. Set aside.
3. In a bowl, whisk together the milk, eggs, onion, red pepper, parsley, red pepper flakes, and black pepper until mixed.
4. Pour the egg mixture into prepared muffin pans.
5. Bake until the muffins are puffed and golden, about 18 to 20 minutes.
6. serve

Nutrition:
Calories 84
Fat 5g
Carbs 3g
Phosphorus 110mg
Potassium 117mg
Sodium 75mg
Protein 7g

Salad with Vinaigrette
Preparation Time: 25 minutes
Cooking Time: 0 minutes
Servings: 4
Ingredients:
For the vinaigrette:

- Caper oil – 1/2 cup
- Balsamic vinegar - 4 Tbsps.
- Chopped fresh oregano – 2 Tbsps.
- Pinch red pepper flakes
- Ground black pepper

For the salad

- Shredded green leaf lettuce – 4 cups
- Carrot – 1, shredded
- Fresh green beans – ¾ cup, cut into 1-inch pieces
- Large radishes – 3, sliced thin

Directions:

1. To make the vinaigrette: put the vinaigrette Ingredients in a bowl and whisk.
2. To make the salad, in a bowl, toss together the carrot, lettuce, green beans, and radishes.

3. Add the vinaigrette to the vegetables and toss to coat.
4. Arrange the salad on plates and serve.

Nutrition:
Calories 273
Fat 27g
Carbs 7g
Phosphorus 30mg
Potassium 197mg
Sodium 27mg
Protein 1g

Salad with Lemon Dressing
Preparation Time: 10 minutes
Cooking Time: 0 minutes
Servings: 4
Ingredients:

- Heavy cream – 1/4 cup
- Freshly squeezed lemon juice – 1/4 cup
- Granulated sugar – 2 Tbsps.
- Chopped fresh dill – 2 Tbsps.
- Finely chopped scallion – 2 Tbsps. green part only
- Ground black pepper – 1/4 tsp.
- English cucumber – 1, sliced thin
- Shredded green cabbage – 2 cups

Directions:
1. In a small bowl, stir together the lemon juice, cream, sugar, dill, scallion, and pepper until well blended.
2. In a large bowl, toss together the cucumber and cabbage.
3. Place the salad in the refrigerator and chill for 1 hour.
4. Stir before serving.

Nutrition:
Calories 99
Fat 6g
Carbs 13g
Phosphorus 38mg
Potassium 200mg
Sodium 14mg
Protein 2g

Shrimp with Salsa
Preparation Time: 15 minutes
Cooking Time: 10 minutes
Servings: 4
Ingredients:

- Caper oil – 2 Tbsp.
- Large shrimp – 6 ounces, peeled and deveined, tails left on
- Minced garlic – 1 tsp.
- Chopped English cucumber – 1/2 cup
- Chopped mango – 1/2 cup
- Zest of 1 lime
- Juice of 1 lime
- Ground black pepper
- Lime wedges for garnish

Directions:
1. Soak 4 wooden skewers in water for 30 minutes.
2. Preheat the barbecue to medium heat.
3. In a bowl, toss together the caper oil, shrimp, and garlic.
4. Thread the shrimp onto the skewers, about 4 shrimp per skewer.
5. In a bowl, stir together the mango, cucumber, lime zest, and lime juice, and season the salsa lightly with pepper. Set aside.
6. Grill the shrimp for 10 minutes, turning once or until the shrimp is opaque and cooked through.
7. Season the shrimp lightly with pepper.
8. Serve the shrimp on the cucumber salsa with lime wedges on the side.

Nutrition:
Calories 120
Fat 8g
Carbs 4g
Phosphorus 91mg
Potassium 129mg
Sodium 60mg
Protein 9g

Pesto Pork Chops

Preparation Time: 20 minutes
Cooking Time: 20 minutes
Servings: 4
Ingredients:

- Pork top-loin chops – 4 (3-ounce) boneless, fat trimmed
- Herb pesto – 8 tsps.
- Breadcrumbs – 1/2 cup
- Caper oil – 1 Tbsp.

Directions:

1. Preheat the oven to 450F.
2. Line a baking sheet with foil. Set aside.
3. Rub 1 tsp. of pesto evenly over both sides of each pork chop.
4. Lightly dredge each pork chop in the breadcrumbs.
5. Heat the oil in a skillet.
6. Brown the pork chops on each side for 5 minutes.
7. Place the pork chops on the baking sheet.
8. Bake for 10 minutes or until pork reaches 145F in the center.

Nutrition:
Calories 210
Fat 7g
Carbs 10g
Phosphorus 179mg
Potassium 220mg
Sodium 148mg
Protein 24g

CHAPTER 6:

Lunch

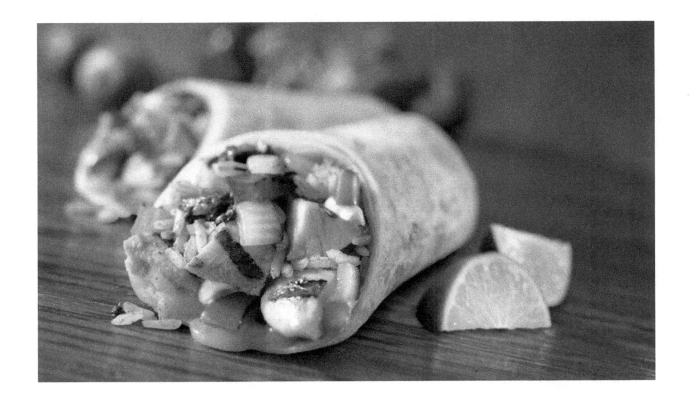

Cucumber Sandwich

Preparation Time: 1 hour
Cooking Time: 5 minutes
Servings: 2
Ingredients:

- 6 tsp. of cream cheese
- 1 pinch of dried dill weed
- 3 tsp. of mayonnaise
- .25 tsp. dry Italian dressing mix
- 4 slices of white bread
- .5 of a cucumber

Directions:

1. Prepare the cucumber and cut it into slices.
2. Mix cream cheese, mayonnaise, and Italian dressing. Chill for one hour.
3. Distribute the mixture onto the white bread slices.
4. Place cucumber slices on top and sprinkle with the dill weed.
5. Cut in halves and serve.

Nutrition:
Calories 143 Fat 6g
Carbs 16.7g Protein 4g
Sodium 255mg Potassium 127mg
Phosphorus 64mg

Pizza Pitas

Preparation Time: 10 minutes
Cooking Time: 10 minutes
Servings: 1
Ingredients:

- .33 cup of mozzarella cheese
- 2 pieces of pita bread, 6 inches in size
- 6 tsp. of chunky red pepper sauce
- 2 cloves of garlic (minced)
- .25 cups of onion, chopped small
- .25 tsp. of red pepper flakes
- .25 cup of bell pepper, chopped small
- 2 ounces of ground pork, lean
- No-stick oil spray
- .5 tsp. of fennel seeds

Directions:

1. Preheat oven to 400.
2. Put the garlic, ground meat, pepper flakes, onion, and bell pepper in a pan. Sauté until cooked.
3. Grease a flat baking pan and put pitas on it. Use the mixture to spread on the pita bread.
4. Spread one tablespoon of the red pepper sauce and top with cheese.
5. Bake for five to eight minutes, until the cheese is bubbling.

Nutrition:
Calories 284 Fat 10g
Carbs 34g Protein 16g
Sodium 795mg Potassium 706mg
Phosphorus 416mg

Lettuce Wraps with Chicken

Preparation Time: 10 minutes
Cooking Time: 15 minutes
Servings: 4
Ingredients:

- 8 lettuce leaves
- .25 cups of fresh cilantro
- .25 cups of mushroom
- 1 tsp. of five spices seasoning
- .25 cups of onion
- 6 tsp. of rice vinegar
- 2 tsp. of hoisin
- 6 tsp. of oil (canola)
- 3 tsp. of oil (sesame)
- 2 tsp. of garlic
- 2 scallions
- 8 ounces of cooked chicken breast

Directions:

1. Mince together the cooked chicken and the garlic. Chop up the onions, cilantro, mushrooms, and scallions.
2. Use a skillet overheat, combine chicken to all remaining ingredients, minus the lettuce leaves. Cook for fifteen minutes, stirring occasionally.
3. Place .25 cups of the mixture into each leaf of lettuce.
4. Wrap the lettuce around like a burrito and eat.

Nutrition:
Calories 84 Fat 4g
Carbs 9g Protein 5.9g
Sodium 618mg Potassium 258mg
Phosphorus 64mg

Turkey Pinwheels

Preparation Time: 10 minutes
Cooking Time: 15 minutes
Servings: 6
Ingredients:

- 6 toothpicks
- 8 oz. of spring mix salad greens
- 1 ten-inch tortilla
- 2 ounces of thinly sliced deli turkey
- 9 tsp. of whipped cream cheese
- 1 roasted red bell pepper

Directions:

1. Cut the red bell pepper into ten strips about a quarter-inch thick.
2. Spread the whipped cream cheese on the tortilla evenly.
3. Add the salad greens to create a base layer and then lay the turkey on top of it.
4. Space out the red bell pepper strips on top of the turkey.
5. Tuck the end and begin rolling the tortilla inward.
6. Use the toothpicks to hold the roll into place and cut it into six pieces.
7. Serve with the swirl facing upward.

Nutrition:
Calories 206 Fat 9g
Carbs 21g
Protein 9g Sodium 533mg
Potassium 145mg
Phosphorus 47mg

Chicken Tacos

Preparation Time: 5 minutes
Cooking Time: 20 minutes
Servings: 4
Ingredients:

- 8 corn tortillas
- 1.5 tsp. of Sodium-free taco seasoning
- 1 juiced lime
- .5 cups of cilantro
- 2 green onions, chopped
- 8 oz. of iceberg or romaine lettuce, shredded or chopped
- .25 cup of sour cream
- 1 pound of boneless and skinless chicken breast

Directions:

1. Cook chicken, by boiling, for twenty minutes. Shred or chop cooked chicken into fine bite-sized pieces.
2. Mix the seasoning and lime juice with the chicken.
3. Put chicken mixture and lettuce in tortillas.
4. Top with the green onions, cilantro, and sour cream.

Nutrition:
Calories 260
Fat 3g
Carbs 36g
Protein 23g
Sodium 122mg
Potassium 445mg
Phosphorus 357mg

Tuna Twist

Preparation Time: 10 minutes
Cooking Time: 30 minutes
Servings: 4
Ingredients:

- 1 can of unsalted or water packaged tuna, drained
- 6 tsp. of vinegar
- .5 cup of cooked peas
- .5 cup celery (chopped)
- 3 tsp. of dried dill weed
- 12 oz. cooked macaroni
- .75 cup of mayonnaise

Directions:

1. Stir together the macaroni, vinegar, and mayonnaise together until blended and smooth.
2. Stir in remaining ingredients.
3. Chill before serving.

Nutrition:
Calories 290
Fat 10g
Carbs 32g
Protein 16g
Sodium 307mg
Potassium 175mg
Phosphorus 111mg

Ciabatta Rolls with Chicken Pesto

Preparation Time: 10 minutes
Cooking Time: 20 minutes
Servings: 2
Ingredients:

- 6 tsp. of Greek yogurt
- 6 tsp. of pesto
- 2 small ciabatta rolls
- 8 oz. of a shredded iceberg or romaine lettuce
- 8 oz. of cooked boneless and skinless chicken breast, shredded
- .125 tsp. of pepper

Directions:

1. Combine the shredded chicken, pesto, pepper, and Greek yogurt in a medium-sized bowl.
2. Slice and toast the ciabatta rolls.
3. Divide the shredded chicken and pesto mixture in half and make sandwiches with the ciabatta rolls.
4. Top with shredded lettuce if desired.

Nutrition:
Calories 374
Fat 10g
Carbs 40g
Protein 30g
Sodium 522mg
Potassium 360mg
Phosphorus 84mg

Marinated Shrimp Pasta Salad

Preparation Time: 15 minutes
Cooking Time: 5 hours
Servings: 1
Ingredients:

- 1/4 cup of honey
- 1/4 cup of balsamic vinegar
- 1/2 of an English cucumber, cubed
- 1/2 pound of fully cooked shrimp
- 15 baby carrots
- 1.5 cups of dime-sized cut cauliflower
- 4 stalks of celery, diced
- 1/2 large yellow bell pepper (diced)
- 1/2 red onion (diced)
- 1/2 large red bell pepper (diced)
- 12 ounces of uncooked tri-color pasta (cooked)
- 3/4 cup of caper oil
- 3 tsp. of mustard (Dijon)
- 1/2 tsp. of garlic (powder)
- 1/2 tsp. pepper

Directions:

1. Cut vegetables and put them in a bowl with the shrimp.
2. Whisk together the honey, balsamic vinegar, garlic powder, pepper, and Dijon mustard in a small bowl. While still whisking, slowly add the oil and whisk it all together.
3. Add the cooked pasta to the bowl with the shrimp and vegetables and mix it.
4. Toss the sauce to coat the pasta, shrimp, and vegetables evenly.
5. Cover and chill for a minimum of five hours before serving. Stir and serve while chilled.

Nutrition:
Calories 205 Fat 13g
Carbs 10g Protein 12g
Sodium 363mg Potassium 156mg
Phosphorus 109mg

Peanut Butter and Jelly Grilled Sandwich

Preparation Time: 5 minutes
Cooking Time: 5 minutes
Servings: 1
Ingredients:

- 2 tsp. butter (unsalted)
- 6 tsp. butter (peanut)
- 3 tsp. of flavored jelly
- 2 pieces of bread

Directions:

1. Put the peanut butter evenly on one bread. Add the layer of jelly.
2. Butter the outside of the pieces of bread.
3. Add the sandwich to a frying pan and toast both sides.

Nutrition:
Calories 300 Fat 7g
Carbs 49g Protein 8g Sodium 460mg
Potassium 222mg Phosphorus 80mg

Grilled Onion and Pepper Jack Grilled Cheese Sandwich

Preparation Time: 5 minutes
Cooking Time: 5 minutes
Servings: 2
Ingredients:
- 1 tsp. of oil (caper)
- 6 tsp. of whipped cream cheese
- 1/2 of a medium onion
- 2 ounces of pepper jack cheese
- 4 slices of rye bread
- 2 tsp. of unsalted butter

Directions:
1. Set out the butter so that it becomes soft. Slice up the onion into thin slices.
2. Sauté onion slices. Continue to stir until cooked. Remove and put it to the side.
3. Spread one tablespoon of the whipped cream cheese on two of the slices of bread.
4. Then add grilled onions and cheese to each slice. Then top using the other two bread slices.
5. Spread the softened butter on the outside of the slices of bread.
6. Use the skillet to toast the sandwiches until lightly brown and the cheese is melted.

Nutrition:
Calories 350
Fat 18g
Carbs 34g
Protein 13g
Sodium 589mg
Potassium 184mg
Phosphorus 226mg

Aromatic Carrot Cream

Preparation Time: 15 minutes
Cooking Time: 25 minutes
Servings: 4
Ingredients:
- 1 tablespoon caper oil
- ½ sweet onion, chopped
- 2 teaspoons fresh ginger, peeled and grated
- 1 teaspoon fresh garlic, minced
- 4 cups water
- 3 carrots, chopped
- 1 teaspoon ground turmeric
- ½ cup coconut milk

Directions:
1. Heat the caper oil into a big pan over medium-high heat.
2. Add the onion, garlic and ginger. Softly cook for about 3 minutes until softened.
3. Include the water, turmeric and the carrots. Softly cook for about 20 minutes (until the carrots are softened).
4. Blend the soup adding coconut milk until creamy.
5. Serve and enjoy!

Nutrition:
Calories 112 Fat 10g
Carbs 8g
Fiber 2g
Protein 2g
Sodium 35mg
Phosphorus 59 mg
Potassium 24mg

Mushrooms Velvet Soup

Preparation Time: 40 minutes
Cooking Time: 40 minutes
Servings: 6
Ingredients:
- 1 teaspoon caper oil
- ½ teaspoon fresh ground black pepper
- 3 medium (85g) shallots, diced
- 2 stalks (80g) celery, chopped
- 1 clove garlic, diced
- 12-ounces cremini mushrooms, sliced
- 5 tablespoons flour
- 4 cups low sodium vegetable stock, divided
- 3 sprigs fresh thyme
- 2 bay leaves
- ½ cup regular yogurt

Directions:

1. Heat oil in a large pan.
2. Add ground pepper, shallots and celery. Cook over medium-high heat.
3. Sauté for 2 minutes until golden.
4. Add garlic and stir.
5. Include the sliced mushrooms. Stir and cook until the mushrooms give out their liquid.
6. Sprawl the flour on the mushrooms and toast for about 2 min.
7. Add one cup of hot stock, thyme sprigs and bay leaves. Stir and add the second cup of stock
8. Stir until well combined.
9. Add the remaining cups of stock.
10. Slowly cook for 15 minutes.
11. Take out bay leaves and thyme sprigs.
12. Blend until mixture is smooth.
13. Include the yogurt and stir well.
14. Slowly cook for 4 minutes.

Serve and enjoy!

Nutrition:
Calories 126
Fat 8g
Carbs 14g
Fiber 2g
Protein 3g
Sodium 108mg
Phosphorus 70mg
Potassium 298mg

Easy Lettuce Wraps

Preparation Time: 15 minutes
Cooking Time: 0 minutes
Servings: 4
Ingredients:

- 8 ounces cooked chicken, shredded
- 1 scallion, chopped
- ½ cup seedless red grapes, halved
- 1 celery stalk, chopped
- ¼ cup mayonnaise
- A pinch ground black pepper
- 4 large lettuce leaves

Directions:

1. In a mixing bowl add the scallion, chicken, celery, grapes and mayonnaise.
2. Stir well until incorporated.
3. Season with pepper.
4. Place the lettuce leaves onto serving plates.
5. Place the chicken salad onto the leaves.
6. Serve and enjoy!

Nutrition:
Calories 146
Fat 5g
Carbs 8g
Fiber 0g
Protein 16g
Sodium 58mg
Phosphorus 125mg
Potassium 212mg

Spaghetti with Pesto

Preparation Time: 10 minutes
Cooking Time: 10 minutes
Servings: 4
Ingredients:

- 8 ounces spaghetti (package pasta)
- 2 cups packed basil leaves
- 2 cups packed arugula leaves
- 1/3 cup walnut pieces
- 3 cloves of garlic
- ¼ cup extra-virgin caper oil
- Black pepper

Directions:

1. Cook pasta with boiling water. Drain.
2. Add the basil, garlic, caper oil, walnuts, pepper and arugula in a blender and mix until creamy.
3. Mix pesto mixture into pasta in a large bowl.
4. Serve and enjoy!

Nutrition:
Calories 400 Fat 21g
Carbs 46g Fiber 3g Protein 11g
Sodium 6mg Phosphorus 113mg
Potassium 202mg

Vegetable Casserole

Preparation Time: 15 minutes
Cooking Time: 15 minutes
Servings: 8
Ingredients:

- 1 teaspoon caper oil
- 1 sweet onion, chopped
- 1 teaspoon garlic, minced
- 2 zucchinis, chopped
- 1 red bell pepper, diced
- 2 carrots, chopped
- 2 cups low-sodium vegetable stock
- 2 large red peppers, chopped
- 2 cups broccoli florets
- 1 teaspoon ground coriander
- ½ teaspoon ground comminutes
- Black pepper

Directions:

1. Heat the caper oil into a big pan over medium-high heat.
2. Add onion and garlic. Softly cook for about 3 minutes until softened.
3. Include the zucchini, carrots, bell pepper and softly cook for 5-6 minutes.
4. Pour the vegetable stock, red peppers, broccoli, coriander, cumin, pepper and stir well.
5. Softly cook for about 5 minutes over medium-high heat until the vegetables are tender.
6. Serve hot and enjoy!

Nutrition:
Calories 47
Fat 1g
Carbs 8 g
Fiber 2g
Protein 2g
Sodium 104mg
Phosphorus 52mg
Potassium 298mg

Appetizing Rice Salad

Preparation Time: 20 minutes
Cooking Time: 1 hour
Servings: 8
Ingredients:

- 1 cup wild rice
- 2 cups water
- 1 tablespoon caper oil
- 2/3 cup walnuts, chopped
- 1 (4 inches) celery rib, sliced
- 4 scallions, thinly sliced
- 2/3 cup raisins
- 1 medium red apple, cored and diced
- ½ cup pomegranate seeds
- ½ tablespoon lemon zest
- 3 tablespoons lemon juice
- Black pepper
- 1/3 cup caper oil

Directions:

1. In a big pot place the wild strained rice together with water and caper oil.
2. Bring to a boil and simmer for about 50 minutes until rice is tender.
3. In a mixing bowl add celery, walnuts, raisins, apple, scallions, pomegranate seeds and lemon zest.
4. Mix well with a blender the lemon juice, pepper, and caper oil.
5. Spread half of this dressing on the apple mixture and mix well.
6. When the rice is cooked, let it cool and incorporate with the fruit mixture
7. Season with the remaining dressing.
8. Serve at room temperature and enjoy!

Nutrition:
Calories 300
Fat 19g
Carbs 34g
Fiber 5g
Protein 6g
Sodium 6mg
Phosphorus 144mg
Potassium 296mg

Spiced Wraps

Preparation Time: 30 minutes
Cooking Time: 0 minutes
Servings: 8
Ingredients:

- 6 ounces cooked chicken breast, minced
- 1 scallion, chopped
- ½ red apple, cored and chopped
- ½ cup bean sprouts
- ¼ cucumber, chopped
- Juice of 1 lime
- Zest of 1 lime
- 2 tablespoons fresh cilantro, chopped
- ½ teaspoon Chinese five-spice powder
- 8 lettuce leaves

Directions:

1. Combine the chicken, apple, bean sprouts, cucumber, lime juice, lime zest, cilantro, five-spice powder and scallions.
2. Place the lettuce leaves onto 8 serving plates.
3. Spoon the chicken mixture onto lettuce leaves.
4. Wrap the lettuce around the chicken mixture.
5. Serve and enjoy!

Nutrition:
Calories 53
Fat 3g
Carbs 3g
Fiber 2g
Protein 7g
Sodium 19mg
Phosphorus 58mg
Potassium 134mg

Rump Roast

Preparation Time: 10 minutes
Cooking Time: 5 hours
Servings: 8
Ingredients:

- 1-pound rump roast
- ½ teaspoon black pepper
- 1 tablespoon caper oil
- ½ small onion, chopped
- 2 teaspoons garlic, minced
- 1 teaspoon dried thyme
- 1 cup + 3 tablespoons water
- 2 tablespoons cornstarch

Directions:

1. Heat the caper oil into a big saucepan over medium heat.
2. Add the peppered meat and brown the roast all over. Set aside the meat.
3. Softly cook the garlic and onion in the same saucepan for about 3 minutes until they are tendered.
4. Incorporate the roast to the saucepan, add 1 cup of water and the thyme.
5. Cover, simmer until the meat is tender or for 4 and half hours.
6. In a mixing bowl, stir the cornstarch with 3 tablespoons water to form a slurry.
7. Beat the slurry into the liquid in the pan and cook for about 15 minutes to thicken the sauce.
8. Serve and enjoy!

Nutrition:
Calories 156
Fat 12g
Carbs 4g
Fiber 0g
Protein 14g
Sodium 48mg
Phosphorus 114mg
Potassium 220mg

Couscous and Sherry Vinaigrette

Preparation Time: 10 minutes
Cooking Time: 30 minutes
Servings: 6
Ingredients:

- For Sherry Vinaigrette: (makes 2/3 cup)
- 2 tablespoons sherry vinegar
- ¼ cup lemon juice
- 1 clove garlic, pressed
- 1/3 cup caper oil

For Roasted Carrots, Cranberries and Couscous:

- 1 medium onion, sliced
- 2 large carrots, sliced
- 2 tablespoons extra-virgin caper oil
- 2 cups pearl couscous
- 2 ½ to 3 cups no sodium vegetable broth
- ½ cup dried cranberries
- ¼ cup Sherry vinaigrette

Directions:

For Sherry Vinaigrette:

1. Beat the vinegar with garlic and lemon juice.
2. Slowly whisk in caper oil.
3. Store refrigerated in a glass jar.

For Carrots, Cranberries and Couscous:

1. Preheat oven to 400°F.
2. Spray a baking dish with cooking spray (caper oil) and place the carrots and onions on it.
3. Roast the vegetables in oven for about 20 minutes until starting to brown. Stir halfway cooking.
4. Heat the couscous in a pan over medium-high heat.
5. Toast the couscous until light brown (about 10 minutes). Stir well.
6. Check the package instructions for the amount of liquid needed for couscous.
7. Bring to a boil the added vegetable stock. Cover and reduce for about 10 minutes. The vegetable stock has to be absorbed.
8. In a mixing bowl, incorporate the couscous with the onions, carrots, cranberries, and sherry vinaigrette. Serve and enjoy!

Nutrition:

Calories 365 Fat 11g
Carbs 58g
Fiber 4g
Protein 9g
Sodium 95mg
Phosphorus 119mg
Potassium 264mg

Crispy Lemon Chicken

Preparation Time: 10 minutes
Cooking Time: 10 minutes
Servings: 4
Ingredients:

- 1 lb. boneless and skinless chicken breast
- ½ cup of all-purpose flour
- 1 large egg
- ½ cup of lemon juice
- 2 tbsp. of water
- ¼ tsp salt
- ¼ tsp lemon pepper
- 1 tsp of mixed herb seasoning
- 2 tbsp. of caper oil
- A few lemon slices for garnishing
- 1 tbsp. of chopped parsley (for garnishing)
- 2 cups of cooked plain white rice

Directions:

1. Slice the chicken breast into thin and season with the herb, salt, and pepper.
2. In a small bowl, whisk together the egg with the water.
3. Keep the flour in a separate bowl.
4. Dip the chicken slices in the egg bath and then into the flour.
5. Heat your oil in a medium frying pan.
6. Shallow fry the chicken in the pan until golden brown.
7. Add the lemon juice and cook for another couple of minutes.
8. Taken the chicken out of the pan and transfer on a wide dish with absorbing paper to absorb any excess oil.
9. Garnish with some chopped parsley and lemon wedges on top.
10. Serve with rice.

Nutrition:

Calories 232
Carbs 24g
Protein 18g
Fat 8g
Sodium 100mg
Potassium 234mg
Phosphorus 217mg

Mexican Steak Tacos

Preparation Time: 10 minutes
Cooking Time: 15 minutes
Servings: 4
Ingredients:

- 1 pound of flank or skirt steak
- ¼ cup of fresh cilantro, chopped
- ¼ cup white onion, chopped
- 3 limes, juiced
- 3 cloves of garlic, minced
- 2 tsp of garlic powder
- 2 tbsp. of caper oil
- ½ cup of Mexican or mozzarella cheese, grated
- 1 tsp of Mexican seasoning
- 8 medium-sized (6") corn flour tortillas

Directions:

1. Combine the juice from two limes, Mexican seasoning, and garlic powder in a dish or bowl and marinate the steak with it for at least half an hour in the fridge.
2. In a separate bowl, combine the chopped cilantro, garlic, onion, and juice from one lime to make your salsa. Cover and keep in the fridge.
3. Slice steak into thin strips and cook for approximately 3 minutes on each side.
4. Preheat your oven to 350F/180C.
5. Distribute evenly the steak strips in each tortilla. Top with a tablespoon of the grated cheese on top.
6. Wrap each taco in aluminum foil and bake in the oven for 7-8 minutes or until cheese is melted.
7. Serve warm with your cilantro salsa.

Nutrition:
Calories 230
Carbs 19.5g
Protein 15g
Fat 11g
Sodium 486.75mg
Potassium 240mg
Phosphorus 268mg

Beer Pork Ribs

Preparation Time: 10 minutes
Cooking Time: 8 hours
Servings: 4
Ingredients:

- 2 pounds of pork ribs, cut into two units/racks
- 18 oz. of root beer
- 2 cloves of garlic, minced
- 2 tbsp. of onion powder
- 2 tbsp. of vegetable oil (optional)

Directions:

1. Wrap the pork ribs with vegetable oil and place one unit on the bottom of your slow cooker with half of the minced garlic and the onion powder.
2. Place the other rack on top with the rest of the garlic and onion powder.
3. Pour over the root beer and cover the lid.
4. Let simmer for 8 hours on low heat.
5. Take off and finish optionally in a grilling pan for a nice sear.

Nutrition:
Calories 301
Carbs 36g
Protein 21g
Fat 18g
Sodium 729mg
Potassium 200mg
Phosphorus 209mg

Mexican Chorizo Sausage

Preparation Time: 10 minutes
Cooking Time: 15 minutes
Servings: 4
Ingredients:

- 2 pounds of boneless pork but coarsely ground
- 3 tbsp. of red wine vinegar
- 2 tbsp. of smoked paprika
- ½ tsp of cinnamon
- ½ tsp of ground cloves
- ¼ tsp of coriander seeds
- ¼ tsp ground ginger
- 1 tsp of ground cumin
- 3 tbsp. of brandy

Directions:

1. In a large mixing bowl, combine the ground pork with the seasonings, brandy, and vinegar and mix with your hands well.
2. Place the mixture into a large Ziploc bag and leave in the fridge overnight.
3. Form into 15-16 patties of equal size.
4. Heat the oil in a large pan and fry the patties for 5-7 minutes on each side, or until the meat inside is no longer pink and there is a light brown crust on top.
5. Serve hot.

Nutrition:

Calories 134
Carbs 0g
Protein: 10g
Fat 7g
Sodium 40 mg
Potassium 138 mg
Phosphorus 128mg

Eggplant Casserole

Preparation Time: 10 minutes
Cooking Time: 25 – 30 minutes
Servings: 4
Ingredients:

- 3 cups of eggplant, peeled and cut into large chunks
- 2 egg whites
- 1 large egg, whole
- ½ cup of unsweetened vegetable
- ¼ tsp of sage
- ½ cup of breadcrumbs
- 1 tbsp. of margarine, melted
- 1/4 tsp garlic salt

Directions:

1. Preheat the oven at 350F/180C.
2. Place the eggplants chunks in a medium pan, cover with a bit of water and cook with the lid covered until tender. Drain from the water and mash with a tool or fork.
3. Beat the eggs with the non-dairy vegetable cream, sage, salt, and pepper. Whisk in the eggplant mush.
4. Combine the melted margarine with the breadcrumbs.

5. Bake in the oven for 20-25 minutes or until the casserole has a golden-brown crust.

Nutrition:

Calories 186 Carbs 19g
Protein 7g Fat 9g
Sodium 503mg
Potassium 230mg
Phosphorus 62mg

Pizza with Chicken and Pesto

Preparation Time: 10 minutes
Cooking Time: 25 minutes
Servings: 4
Ingredients:

- 1 ready-made frozen pizza dough
- 2/3 cup cooked chicken, chopped
- 1/2 cup of orange bell pepper, diced
- 1/2 cup of green bell pepper, diced
- 1/4 cup of purple onion, chopped
- 2 tbsp. of green basil pesto
- 1 tbsp. of chives, chopped
- 1/3 cup of parmesan or Romano cheese, grated
- 1/4 cup of mozzarella cheese
- 1 tbsp. of caper oil

Directions:

1. Thaw the pizza dough according to instructions on the package.
2. Heat the caper oil in a pan and sauté the peppers and onions for a couple of minutes. Set aside
3. Once the pizza dough has thawed, spread the Bali pesto over its surface.
4. Top with half of the cheese, the peppers, the onions, and the chicken. Finish with the rest of the cheese.
5. Bake at 350F/180C for approx. 20 minutes (or until crust and cheese are baked).
6. Slice in triangles with a pizza cutter or sharp knife and serve.

Nutrition:

Calories 225 Carbs 13.9g Protein 11.1g
Fat 12g Sodium 321mg Potassium 174mg
Phosphorus 172mg

Shrimp Quesadilla
Preparation Time: 10 minutes
Cooking Time: 10 minutes
Servings: 2
Ingredients:
- 5 oz. of shrimp, shelled and deveined
- 4 tbsp. of Mexican salsa
- 2 tbsp. of fresh cilantro, chopped
- 1 tbsp. of lemon juice
- 1 tsp of ground cumin
- 1 tsp of cayenne pepper
- 2 tbsp. of unsweetened soy yogurt or creamy tofu
- 2 medium corn flour tortillas
- 2 tbsp. of low-fat cheddar cheese

Directions:
1. Mix the cilantro, cumin, lemon juice, and cayenne in a Ziploc bag to make your marinade.
2. Put the shrimps and marinate for 10 minutes.
3. Heat a pan over medium heat with some caper oil and toss in the shrimp with the marinade. Let cook for a couple of minutes or as soon as shrimps have turned pink and opaque.
4. Add the soy cream or soft tofu to the pan and mix well. Remove from the heat and keep the marinade aside.
5. Heat tortillas in the grill or microwave for a few seconds.
6. Place 2 tbsp. of salsa on each tortilla. Top one tortilla with the shrimp mixture and add the cheese on top.
7. Stack one tortilla against each other (with the spread salsa layer facing the shrimp mixture).
8. Transfer this on a baking tray and cook for 7-8 minutes at 350F/180C to melt the cheese and crisp up the tortillas.
9. Serve warm.

Nutrition:
Calories 255 Carbs 21g
Fat 9g Protein 24g
Sodium 562mg Potassium 235mg
Phosphorus 189mg

Grilled Corn on the Cob
Preparation Time: 5 minutes
Cooking Time: 20 minutes
Servings: 4
Ingredients:
- 4 frozen corn on the cob, cut in half
- ½ tsp of thyme
- 1 tbsp. of grated parmesan cheese
- ¼ tsp of black pepper

Directions:
1. Combine the oil, cheese, thyme, and black pepper in a bowl.
2. Place the corn in the cheese/oil mix and roll to coat evenly.
3. Fold all 4 pieces in aluminum foil, leaving a small open surface on top.
4. Place the wrapped corns over the grill and let cook for 20 minutes.
5. Serve hot.

Nutrition:
Calories 125
Carbs 29.5g
Protein 2g
Fat 1.3g
Sodium 26mg
Potassium 145mg
Phosphorus 91.5mg

Couscous with Veggies
Preparation Time: 10 minutes
Cooking Time: 10 minutes
Servings: 5
Ingredients:
- ½ cup of uncooked couscous
- ¼ cup of white mushrooms, sliced
- ½ cup of red onion, chopped
- 1 garlic clove, minced
- ½ cup of frozen peas
- 2 tbsp. of dry white wine
- ½ tsp of basil
- 2 tbsp. of fresh parsley, chopped
- 1 cup water or vegetable stock
- 1 tbsp. of margarine or vegetable oil

Directions:
1. Thaw the peas by setting them aside at room temperature for 15-20 minutes.

2. In a medium pan, heat the margarine or vegetable oil.

3. Add the onions, peas, mushroom, and garlic and sauté for around 5 minutes. Add the wine and let it evaporate.

4. Add all the herbs and spices and toss well. Take off the heat and keep aside.

5. In a small pot, cook the couscous with 1 cup of hot water or vegetable stock. Bring to a boil, take off the heat, and sit for a few minutes with a lid covered.

6. Add the sauté veggies to the couscous and toss well.

7. Serve in a serving bowl warm or cold.

Nutrition:

Calories 110.4

Carbs18g

Protein 3g

Fat 2g

Sodium 112.2mg

Potassium 69.6mg

Phosphorus 46.8mg

Easy Egg Salad

Preparation Time: 5 minutes

Cooking Time: 8 minutes

Servings: 4

Ingredients:

- 4 large eggs
- ½ cup of sweet onion, chopped
- ¼ cup of celery, chopped
- 2 tbsp. of pickle relish
- 1 tbsp. of yellow mustard
- 1 tsp of smoked paprika
- 3 tbsp. of mayo

Directions:

1. Hard boil the eggs in a small pot filled with water for approx. 7-8 minutes. Leave the eggs in the water for an extra couple of minutes before peeling.

2. Peel the eggs and chop finely with a knife or tool.

3. Combine all the chopped veggies with the mayo and mustard. Add in the eggs and mix well.

4. Sprinkle with some smoked paprika on top.

5. Serve cold with pitta, white bread slices, or lettuce wraps.

Nutrition:

Calories 127

Carbs 6g

Protein 7g

Fat 13g

Sodium 170.7mg

Potassium 87.5mg

Phosphorus 101mg

CHAPTER 7:

Dinner

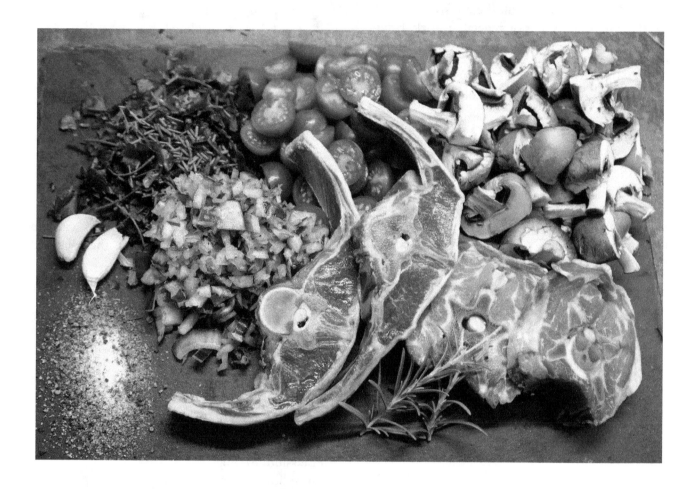

Lemon and Broccoli Platter

Preparation Time: 10 minutes
Cooking Time: 15 minutes
Servings: 6
Ingredients:

- 2 heads broccoli, separated into florets
- 2 teaspoons extra virgin caper oil
- 1 teaspoon salt
- 1/2 teaspoon black pepper
- 1 garlic clove, minced
- 1/2 teaspoon lemon juice

Directions:

1. Preheat your oven to 400 °F
2. Take a large-sized bowl and add broccoli florets
3. Drizzle caper oil and season with pepper, salt, and garlic
4. Spread the broccoli out in a single even layer on a baking sheet
5. Bake for 15-20 minutes until fork tender
6. Squeeze lemon juice on top
7. Serve and enjoy!

Nutrition:
Calories 49
Fat 1.9g
Carbs 7g
Protein 3g
Phosphorus 12mg
Potassium 32mg
Sodium 22 mg

Chicken Liver Stew

Preparation Time: 10 minutes
Cooking Time: 20 minutes
Servings: 2
Ingredients:

- 10 ounces chicken livers
- 1-ounce onion, chopped
- 2 ounces sour cream
- 1 tablespoon caper oil
- Salt to taste

Directions:

1. Take a pan and place it over medium heat

2. Add oil and let it heat up
3. Add onions and fry until just browned
4. Add livers and season with salt
5. Cook until livers are half cooked
6. Transfer the mix to a stew pot
7. Add sour cream and cook for 20 minutes
8. Serve and enjoy!

Nutrition:
Calories 146 Fat 9g
Carbs 2g
Phosphorus 12mg
Potassium 32mg
Sodium 22 mg
Protein 15g

Simple Lamb Chops

Preparation Time: 35 minutes
Cooking Time: 5 minutes
Servings: 3
Ingredients:

- 1/4 cup caper oil
- 1/4 cup mint, fresh and chopped
- 8 lamb rib chops
- 1 tablespoon garlic, minced
- 1 tablespoon rosemary, fresh and chopped

Directions:

1. Add rosemary, garlic, mint, caper oil into a bowl and mix well
2. Keep a tablespoon of the mixture on the side for later use
3. Toss lamb chops into the marinade, letting them marinate for 30 minutes
4. Take a cast-iron skillet and place it over medium-high heat
5. Add lamb and cook for 2 minutes per side for medium-rare
6. Let the lamb rest for a few minutes and drizzle the remaining marinade
7. Serve and enjoy!

Nutrition:
Calories 566 Fat 40g Carbs 2g
Protein 47g Phosphorus 12mg
Potassium 32mg Sodium 22mg

Chicken and Mushroom Stew

Preparation Time: 10 minutes
Cooking Time: 35 minutes
Servings: 4
Ingredients:

- 4 chicken breast halves, cut into bite-sized pieces
- 1-pound mushrooms, sliced (5-6 cups)
- 1 bunch spring onion, chopped
- 4 tablespoons caper oil
- 1 teaspoon thyme
- Salt and pepper as needed

Directions:

1. Take a large deep-frying pan and place it over medium-high heat
2. Add oil and let it heat up
3. Add chicken and cook for 4-5 minutes per side until slightly browned
4. Add spring onions and mushrooms, season with salt and pepper according to your taste
5. Stir
6. Cover with lid and bring the mix to a boil
7. Lower heat and simmer for 25 minutes
8. Serve!

Nutrition:
Calories 247 Fat 12g
Carbs 10g
Phosphorus 12mg
Potassium 32mg
Sodium 22 mg
Protein 23g

Roasted Carrot Soup

Preparation Time: 10 minutes
Cooking Time: 50 minutes
Servings: 4
Ingredients:

- 8 large carrots, washed and peeled
- 6 tablespoons caper oil
- 1-quart broth
- Cayenne pepper to taste
- Salt and pepper to taste

Directions:

1. Preheat your oven to 425 °F
2. Take a baking sheet and add carrots, drizzle caper oil and roast for 30-45 minutes
3. Put roasted carrots into a blender and add the broth, puree
4. Pour into saucepan and heat soup
5. Season with salt, pepper, and cayenne
6. Drizzle caper oil
7. Serve and enjoy!

Nutrition:
Calories 222 Fat 18g
Phosphorus 12mg Potassium 32mg
Sodium 22 mgCarbs 7g Protein 5g

Garlic and Butter-Flavored Cod

Preparation Time: 5 minutes
Cooking Time: 20 minutes
Servings: 3
Ingredients:

- 3 Cod fillets, 8 ounces each
- ¾ pound baby bok choy halved
- 1/3 cup almond butter, thinly sliced
- 1 1/2 tablespoons garlic, minced
- Salt and pepper to taste

Directions:

1. Preheat your oven to 400 °F
2. Cut 3 sheets of aluminum foil (large enough to fit fillet)
3. Place cod fillet on each sheet and add butter and garlic on top
4. Add bok choy, season with pepper and salt
5. Fold packet and enclose them in pouches
6. Arrange on baking sheet
7. Bake for 20 minutes
8. Transfer to a cooling rack and let them cool   Enjoy!

Nutrition:
Calories 355 Fat 21g
Phosphorus 12mg
Potassium 32mgSodium 22 mg
Carbs 3g Protein 37g

Tilapia Broccoli Platter

Preparation Time: 4 minutes
Cooking Time: 14 minutes
Servings: 2
Ingredients:

- 6 ounces of tilapia, frozen
- 1 tablespoon of almond butter
- 1 tablespoon of garlic, minced
- 1 teaspoon of lemon pepper seasoning
- 1 cup of broccoli florets, fresh

Directions:

1. Preheat your oven to 350 °F
2. Add fish in aluminum foil packets
3. Arrange the broccoli around fish
4. Sprinkle lemon pepper on top
5. Close the packets and seal
6. Bake for 14 minutes
7. Take a bowl and add garlic and butter, mix well and keep the mixture on the side
8. Remove the packet from the oven and transfer to a platter
9. Place butter on top of the fish and broccoli, serve and enjoy!

Nutrition:
Calories 362
Fat 25g
Carbs 2g
Protein 29g

Parsley Scallops

Preparation Time: 5 minutes
Cooking Time: 25 minutes
Servings: 4
Ingredients:

- 8 tablespoons almond butter
- 2 garlic cloves, minced
- 16 large sea scallops
- Salt and pepper to taste
- 1 1/2 tablespoons caper oil

Directions:

1. Seasons scallops with salt and pepper

2. Take a skillet and place it over medium heat, add oil and let it heat up
3. Sauté scallops for 2 minutes per side, repeat until all scallops are cooked
4. Add butter to the skillet and let it melt
5. Stir in garlic and cook for 15 minutes
6. Return scallops to skillet and stir to coat
7. Serve and enjoy!

Nutrition:
Calories 417
Phosphorus: 12mg
Potassium 32mg
Sodium 22 mg
Fat 31g
Carbs 5g
Protein 29g

Blackened Chicken

Preparation Time: 10 minutes
Cooking Time: 10 minutes
Servings: 4
Ingredients:

- 1/2 teaspoon paprika
- 1/8 teaspoon salt
- 1/4 teaspoon cayenne pepper
- 1/4 teaspoon ground cumin
- 1/4 teaspoon dried thyme
- 1/8 teaspoon ground white pepper
- 1/8 teaspoon onion powder
- 2 chicken breasts, boneless and skinless

Directions:

1. Preheat your oven to 350 °F
2. Grease baking sheet
3. Take a cast-iron skillet and place it over high heat
4. Add oil and heat it up for 5 minutes until smoking hot
5. Take a small bowl and mix salt, paprika, cumin, white pepper, cayenne, thyme, onion powder

6. Oil the chicken breast on both sides and coat the breast with the spice mix
7. Transfer to your hot pan and cook for 1 minute per side
8. Transfer to your prepared baking sheet and bake for 5 minutes
9. Serve and enjoy!

Nutrition:
Calories 136
Fat 3g
Carbs 1g
Phosphorus 12mg
Potassium 32mg
Sodium 22 mg
Protein 24g

Spicy Paprika Lamb Chops

Preparation Time: 10 minutes
Cooking Time: 15 minutes
Servings: 4
Ingredients:

- 2 lamb racks, cut into chops
- Salt and pepper to taste
- 3 tablespoons paprika
- ¾ cup cumin powder
- 1 teaspoon chili powder

Directions:

1. Take a bowl and add the paprika, cumin, chili, salt, pepper, and stir
2. Add lamb chops and rub the mixture
3. Heat grill over medium-temperature and add lamb chops, cook for 5 minutes
4. Flip and cook for 5 minutes more, flip again
5. Cook for 2 minutes, flip and cook for 2 minutes more
6. Serve and enjoy!

Nutrition:
Calories 200
Fat 5g
Phosphorus 12mg
Potassium 32mg
Sodium 22 mg
Carbs 4g
Protein 8g

Mushroom and Caper Sirloin Steak

Preparation Time: 10 minutes
Cooking Time: 14 minutes
Servings: 4
Ingredients:

- 1-pound boneless beef sirloin steak, ¾ inch thick, cut into 4 pieces
- 1 large red onion, chopped
- 1 cup mushrooms
- 4 garlic cloves, thinly sliced
- 4 tablespoons caper oil
- 1/2 cup green capers, coarsely chopped
- 1 cup parsley leaves, finely cut

Directions:

1. Take a large-sized skillet and place it over medium-high heat
2. Add oil and let it heat p
3. Add beef and cook until both sides are browned, remove beef and drain fat
4. Add the rest of the oil to skillet and heat it up
5. Add onions, garlic and cook for 2-3 minutes
6. Stir well
7. Add mushrooms capers and cook until mushrooms are thoroughly done
8. Return beef to skillet and lower heat to medium
9. Cook for 3-4 minutes (covered)
10. Stir in parsley
11. Serve and enjoy!

Nutrition:
Calories 386
Fat 30g
Carbs 11g
Phosphorus 12mg
Potassium 32mg
Sodium 22 mg
Protein 21g

Parsley and Chicken Breast

Preparation Time: 10 minutes
Cooking Time: 40 minutes
Servings: 4
Ingredients:

- 1 tablespoon dry parsley
- 1 tablespoon dry basil
- 4 chicken breast halves, boneless and skinless
- 1/2 teaspoon salt
- 1/2 teaspoon red pepper flakes, crushed

Directions:

1. Preheat your oven to 350 °F
2. Take a 9x13 inch baking dish and grease it with cooking spray
3. Sprinkle 1 tablespoon of parsley, 1 teaspoon of basil and spread the mixture over your baking dish
4. Arrange the chicken breast halves over the dish and sprinkle garlic slices on top
5. Take a small bowl and add 1 teaspoon parsley, 1 teaspoon of basil, salt, basil, red pepper and mix well. Pour the mixture over the chicken breast
6. Bake for 25 minutes
7. Remove the cover and bake for 15 minutes more Serve and enjoy!

Nutrition:
Calories 150 Fat 4g Carbs 4g
Phosphorus 112mg Potassium 132mg
Sodium 222mg Protein 25g

Simple Mustard Chicken

Preparation Time: 10 minutes
Cooking Time: 40 minutes
Servings: 4
Ingredients:

- 4 chicken breasts
- 1/2 cup chicken broth
- 3-4 tablespoons mustard
- 3 tablespoons caper oil
- 1 teaspoon paprika
- 1 teaspoon chili powder
- 1 teaspoon garlic powder

Directions:

1. Take a small bowl and mix mustard, caper oil, paprika, chicken broth, garlic powder, chicken broth, and chili
2. Add chicken breast and marinate for 30 minutes
3. Take a lined baking sheet and arrange the chicken
4. Bake for 35 minutes at 375 °F
5. Serve and enjoy!

Nutrition:
Calories 531
Fat 23g
Phosphorus: 112mg
Potassium 132mg
Sodium 222mg
Carbs 10g
Protein 64g

CHAPTER 8:

Drinks and Smoothies

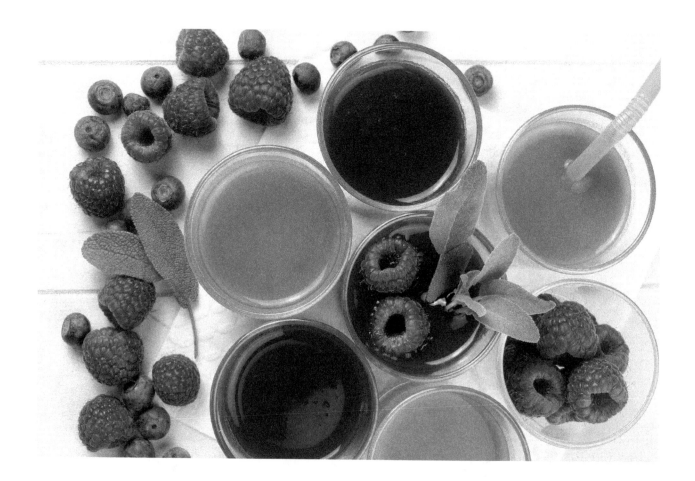

Fruity Smoothie

Preparation Time: 10minutes
Cooking Time: 0 minutes
Servings: 2
Ingredients:

- 8 oz. canned fruits, with juice
- 2 scoops vanilla-flavored whey protein powder
- 1 cup cold water
- 1 cup crushed ice

Directions:

1. First, start by putting all the ingredients in a blender jug.
2. Give it a pulse for 30 seconds until blended well.
3. Serve chilled and fresh.

Nutrition:

Calories 186 Protein 23g
Fat 2g Phosphorus: 112mg
Potassium 132mg
Sodium 222mg
Fiber 1.1g

Mixed Berry Protein Smoothie

Preparation Time: 10minutes
Cooking Time: 0 minutes
Servings: 2
Ingredients:

- 4 oz. cold water
- 1 cup frozen mixed berries
- 2 ice cubes
- 1 tsp blueberry essence
- 1/2 cup whipped cream topping
- 2 scoops whey protein powder

Directions:

1. First, start by putting all the ingredients in a blender jug.
2. Give it a pulse for 30 seconds until blended well.
3. Serve chilled and fresh.

Nutritional:

Calories 104 Protein 6g
Fat 4g
Phosphorus: 112mg
Potassium 132mg
Sodium 222mg
Fiber 2.4g

Peach High-Protein Smoothie

Preparation Time: 10minutes
Cooking Time: 0 minutes
Servings: 1
Ingredients:

- 1/2 cup ice
- 2 tbsp. powdered egg whites
- 3/4 cup fresh peaches
- 1 tbsp. sugar

Directions:

1. First, start by putting all the ingredients in a blender jug.
2. Give it a pulse for 30 seconds until blended well.
3. Serve chilled and fresh.

Nutrition:

Calories 132
Protein 10g
Fat 0g
Phosphorus: 112mg
Potassium 132mg
Sodium 222mg
Fiber 1.9g

Strawberry Fruit Smoothie

Preparation Time: 10minutes
Cooking Time: 0 minutes
Servings: 1
Ingredients:

- 3/4 cup fresh strawberries
- 1/2 cup liquid pasteurized egg whites
- 1/2 cup ice
- 1 tbsp. sugar

Directions:

1. First, start by putting all the ingredients in a blender jug.
2. Give it a pulse for 30 seconds until blended well.
3. Serve chilled and fresh.

Nutrition:

Calories 156
Protein 14g
Fat 0g
Phosphorus: 112mg
Potassium 132mg
Sodium 222mg
Fiber 2.5g

Watermelon Bliss

Preparation Time: 10minutes
Cooking Time: 0 minutes
Servings: 2
Ingredients:

- 2 cups watermelon
- 1 medium-sized cucumber, peeled and sliced
- 2 mint sprigs, leaves only
- 1 celery stalk
- Squeeze of lime juice

Directions:

1. First, start by putting all the ingredients in a blender jug.
2. Give it a pulse for 30 seconds until blended well.
3. Serve chilled and fresh.

Nutrition:
Calories 156
Protein 14g
Fat 0 g
Phosphorus: 112mg
Potassium 132mg
Sodium 222mg
Fiber 2.5g

Cranberry Smoothie

Preparation Time: 10minutes
Cooking Time: 0 minutes
Servings: 1
Ingredients:

- 1 cup frozen cranberries
- 1 medium cucumber, peeled and sliced
- 1 stalk of celery
- Handful of parsley
- Squeeze of lime juice

Directions:

1. First, start by putting all the ingredients in a blender jug. Give it a pulse for 30 seconds until blended well.
2. Serve chilled and fresh.

Nutrition:
Calories 126 Protein 12g
Fat 0.03g Phosphorus: 112mg
Potassium 132mg
Sodium 222mg Fiber 1.4g

Berry Cucumber Smoothie

Preparation Time: 10minutes
Cooking Time: 0 minutes
Servings: 1
Ingredients:

- 1 medium cucumber, peeled and sliced
- ½ cup fresh blueberries
- ½ cup fresh or frozen strawberries
- ½ cup unsweetened rice milk
- Stevia, to taste

Directions:

1. First, start by putting all the ingredients in a blender jug.
2. Give it a pulse for 30 seconds until blended well.
3. Serve chilled and fresh.

Nutrition:
Calories 141
Protein 10g
Carbs 15g
Fat 0g
Sodium 113mg
Potassium 230mg
Phosphorus 129mg

Raspberry Peach Smoothie

Preparation Time: 10minutes
Cooking Time: 0 minutes
Servings: 2
Ingredients:

- 1 cup frozen raspberries
- 1 medium peach, pit removed, sliced
- ½ cup silken tofu
- 1 tbsp. honey
- 1 cup unsweetened vanilla almond milk

Directions:

1. First, start by putting all the ingredients in a blender jug.
2. Give it a pulse for 30 seconds until blended well.
3. Serve chilled and fresh.

Nutrition:
Calories 132 Protein 9g
Carbs 14g Sodium 112mg
Potassium 310mg Phosphorus 39mg

Power-Boosting Smoothie

Preparation Time: 5 minutes
Cooking Time: 0 minutes
Servings: 2
Ingredients:

- ½ cup water
- ½ cup non-dairy whipped topping
- 2 scoops whey protein powder
- 1½ cups frozen blueberries

Directions:

1. In a high-speed blender, add all ingredients and pulse till smooth.
2. Transfer into 2 serving glass and serve immediately.

Nutrition:

Calories 242
Fat 7g
Carbs 23.8g
Protein 23.2g
Potassium 263mg
Sodium 63mg
Phosphorous 30mg

Distinctive Pineapple Smoothie

Preparation Time: 5 minutes
Cooking Time: 0 minutes
Servings: 2
Ingredients:

- ¼ cup crushed ice cubes
- 2 scoops vanilla whey protein powder
- 1 cup water
- 1½ cups pineapple

Directions:

1. In a high-speed blender, add all ingredients and pulse till smooth.
2. Transfer into 2 serving glass and serve immediately.

Nutrition:

Calories 117
Fat 2.1g
Carbs 18.2g
Protein 22.7g
Potassium 296mg
Sodium 81mg
Phosphorous 28mg

Strengthening Smoothie Bowl

Preparation Time: 5 minutes
Cooking Time: 4 minutes
Servings: 2
Ingredients:

- ¼ cup fresh blueberries
- ¼ cup fat-free plain Greek yogurt
- 1/3 cup unsweetened almond milk
- 2 tbsp. of whey protein powder
- 2 cups frozen blueberries

Directions:

1. In a blender, add blueberries and pulse for about 1 minute.
2. Add almond milk, yogurt and protein powder and pulse till desired consistency.
3. Transfer the mixture into 2 bowls evenly.
4. Serve with the topping of fresh blueberries.

Nutrition:

Calories 176
Fat 2.1g
Carbs 27g
Protein 15.1g
Potassium 242mg
Sodium 72mg
Phosphorous 555.3mg

Pineapple Juice

Preparation Time: 5 minutes
Cooking Time: 0 minutes
Servings: 2
Ingredients:

- ½ cup canned pineapple
- 1 cup water

Direction:

1. Blend all ingredients and serve over ice.

Nutrition:

Calories 41
Protein 0g
Carbs 11g
Fat 0g
Sodium 0.4mg
Potassium 180mg
Phosphorus 8mg

Grapefruit Sorbet

Preparation Time: 10 minutes
Cooking Time: 5 minutes
Servings: 6
Ingredients

- ½ cup sugar
- ¼ cup water
- 1 fresh thyme sprig
- For the sorbet
- Juice of 6 pink grapefruit
- ¼ cup thyme simple syrup

Directions:

1 In a blender, combine the grapefruit juice and ¼ cup of simple syrup, and process.
2 Transfer to an airtight container and freeze for 3 to 4 hours, until firm. Serve.
3 Substitution tip: Try this with other citrus fruits, such as lemons, or limes, for an equally delicious treat.

Nutrition:
Calories 117 Fat 2.1g
Carbs 18.2g
Protein 22.7g
Potassium 296mg
Sodium 81mg
Phosphorous 28mg

Apple and Blueberry Crisp

Preparation Time: 1 hour 10 minutes
Cooking Time: 1 hour
Serving: 8
Ingredients:

- Crisp
- 1/4 cup of brown sugar
- 1 1/4 cups quick cooking rolled oats
- 6 tbsp. non-hydrogenated melted margarine
- 1/4 cup all-purpose flour (unbleached)

Filling:

- 2 tbsp. cornstarch
- 1/2 cup of brown sugar
- 2 cups chopped or grated apples
- cups frozen or fresh blueberries (not thawed)
- 1 tbsp. fresh lemon juice
- 1 tbsp. melted margarine

Directions:

1 Preheat the oven to 350°F with the rack in the middle position.
2 Pour all the dry ingredients into a bowl, then the butter and stir until it is moistened. Set the mixture aside.
3 In an 8-inch (20-cm) square baking dish, mix the cornstarch and brown sugar. Add lemon juice and the rest of the fruits. Toss to blend the mixture. Add the crisp mixture, then bake until the crisp turns golden brown (or for 55 minutes to 1 hour). You can either serve cold or warm.

Nutrition:
Calories 127
Fat 2.1g
Carbs 18.2g
Protein 22.7g
Potassium 256mg
Sodium 61mg
Phosphorous 28mg

Mini Pineapple Upside Down Cakes

Preparation Time: 50 minutes
Cooking Time: 50 minutes
Servings: 12
Ingredients:

- 1 tbsp. melted unsalted butter
- 12 canned unsweetened pineapple slices
- 1/3 cup packed brown sugar
- 2/3 cup sugar
- fresh cherries cut into halves and pitted
- 1 tbsp. canola oil
- 2/3 cup milk (fat-free)
- ½ tbsp. lemon juice
- 1 large egg
- 1-1/3 cups cake flour
- 1/4 tbsp. vanilla extract
- 1/4 tsp salt
- 1-1/4 tsp baking powder

Directions:

1 Coat 12 serving muffin pan with butter or you could use a square baking pan.
2 Sprinkle little brown sugar into each of the sections.

3   Crush 1 pineapple slice into each section to take the shape of the cup. Place 1 half cherry in the center of the pineapple with the cut side facing up.

4   Get a large bowl and beat the egg, milk, and the extracts until it is evenly blended.

5   Beat the flour, salt, and baking powder into sugar mixture until it is well blended to attain homogeneity and pour it into the batter prepared in the muffin pan.

6   Bake at 350°s until a toothpick sinks in and comes out clean (or for 35-40 minutes). Invert the muffin pan immediately and allow the cooked cakes to drop onto a serving plate. (If necessary, you can use a small spatula or butter knife to gently release them from the pan.)

7   Serve warm.

Nutrition:
Calories 119
Fat 2.1g
Carbs 16.2g
Protein 22.7g
Potassium 296mg
Sodium 81mg
Phosphorous 28mg

CHAPTER 9:

Snacks

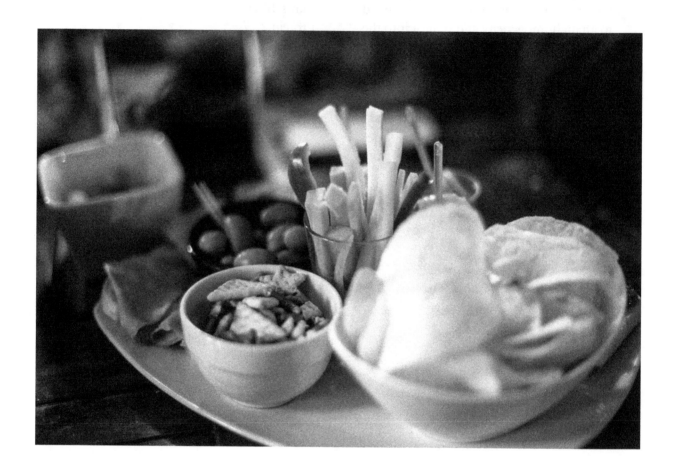

Popcorn with Sugar and Spice

Preparation Time: 10 minutes
Cooking Time: 10 minutes
Servings: 2
Ingredients:

- 8 cups hot popcorn
- 2 tablespoons unsalted butter
- 2 tablespoons sugar
- 1/2 teaspoon cinnamon
- 1/4 teaspoon nutmeg

Directions:

1. Popping the corn; put aside.
2. Heat the butter, sugar, cinnamon, and nutmeg in the microwave or saucepan over a range fire until the butter is melted, and the sugar dissolved.
3. Sprinkle the corn with the spicy butter, mix well.
4. Serve immediately for optimal flavor.

Nutrition:

Calories 120
Fat 7g
Carbs 12g
Protein 2g
Sodium 2mg
Potassium 56mg
Phosphorus 60mg

Eggplant and Chickpea Bites

Preparation Time: 15 minutes
Cooking Time: 50 minutes
Servings: 6
Ingredients:

- 3 large eggplants cut in half (make a few cuts in the flesh with a knife)
- 2 large cloves garlic, peeled and deglazed
- 2 tbsp. coriander powder
- 2 tbsp. cumin seeds
- 400 g canned chickpeas, rinsed and drained
- 2 Tbsp. chickpea flour
- Zest and juice of 1/2 lemon
- 1/2 lemon quartered for serving
- 3 tbsp. tablespoon of polenta

Directions:

1. Heat the oven to 200°C. Spray the eggplant halves generously with oil and place them on the meat side up on a baking sheet.
2. Sprinkle with coriander and cumin seeds, and then place the cloves of garlic on the plate.
3. Season and roast for 40 minutes until the flesh of eggplant is completely tender. Reserve and let cool a little.
4. Scrape the flesh of the eggplant in a bowl with a spatula and throw the skins in the compost. Thoroughly scrape and make sure to incorporate spices and crushed roasted garlic.
5. Add chickpeas, chickpea flour, zest, and lemon juice. Crush roughly and mix well.
6. Check to season. Do not worry if the mixture seems a bit soft - it will firm up in the fridge.
7. Form about twenty pellets and place them on a baking sheet covered with parchment paper. Refrigerate for at least 30 minutes.
8. Preheat oven to 180°C. Remove the meatballs from the fridge and coat them by rolling them in the polenta.
9. Place them back on the baking sheet and spray a little oil on each. Roast for 20 minutes until golden and crisp.
10. Serve with lemon wedges. You can also serve these dumplings with a spicy yogurt dip.

Nutrition:

Calories 72 Fat 1g
Carbs 18g
Protein 3g
Sodium 63mg
Potassium 162mg
Phosphorus 36mg

Baba Ghanouj

Preparation Time: 10 minutes
Cooking Time: 1 hour and 20 minutes
Servings: 1
Ingredients:

- 1 large eggplant, cut in half lengthwise
- 1 head of garlic, unpeeled
- 30 ml (2 tablespoons) of caper oil
- Lemon juice to taste

Directions:

1. Preheat the oven to 350 degrees F.
2. Place the eggplant on the plate, skin side up. Roast until the meat is very tender and detaches easily from the skin, about 1 hour depending on the eggplant's size. Let cool.
3. Meanwhile, cut the tip of the garlic cloves. Put garlic cloves in a square aluminum foil. Fold the edges of the sheet and fold together to form a tightly wrapped foil.
4. Roast with the eggplant until tender, about 20 minutes. Let cool. Purée the pods with a garlic press.
5. With a spoon, scoop out the eggplant's flesh and place it in the bowl of a food processor. Add the garlic puree, the oil, and the lemon juice. Stir until purée is smooth and pepper.
6. Serve with mini pita bread.

Nutrition:

Calories 110 Fat 12g
Carbs 5g Protein 1g
Sodium 180mg Potassium 207mg
Phosphorus 81mg

Baked Pita Chips

Preparation Time: 5 minutes
Cooking Time: 15 minutes
Servings: 6
Ingredients:

- 3 pita loaves (6 inches)
- 3 tablespoons caper oil
- Chili powder

Directions:

1. Separate each bread in half with scissors to obtain 6 round pieces.
2. Cut each piece into eight points. Brush each with caper oil and sprinkle with chili powder.
3. Bake at 350 degrees F for about 15 minutes until crisp.

Nutrition:

Calories 120 Fat 2.5g
Carbs 22g Protein 3g
Sodium 70mg Potassium 0mg
Phosphorus 0mg

Herbal Cream Cheese Tartines

Preparation Time: 15 minutes
Cooking Time: 15 minutes
Servings: 2
Ingredients:

- 20 regular round melba crackers
- 1 clove garlic, halved
- 1 cup cream cheese spread
- ¼ cup chopped herbs such as chives, dill, parsley, tarragon, or thyme
- 2 tbsp. minced French shallot or onion
- ½ tsp. black pepper
- 2 tbsp. tablespoons water

Directions:

1. In a medium-sized bowl, combine the cream cheese, herbs, shallot, pepper, and water with a hand blender.
2. Rub the crackers with the cut side of the garlic clove.
3. Serve the cream cheese with the rusks.

Nutrition:

Calories 476
Fat 9g
Carbs 75g
Protein 23g
Sodium 885mg
Potassium 312mg
Phosphorus 165mg

Mixes of Snacks

Preparation Time: 15 minutes
Cooking Time: 1 hour
Servings: 1
Ingredients:

- 6 c. margarine
- 2 tbsp. Worcestershire sauce
- 1 ½ tbsp. spice salt
- ¾ c. garlic powder
- ½ tsp. onion powder
- 3 cups Cheerios
- 3 cups corn flakes
- 1 cup pretzel
- 1 cup broken bagel chip into 1-inch pieces

Directions:

1. Preheat the oven to 250F (120C)
2. Melt the margarine in a large roasting pan. Stir in the seasoning. Gradually add the

ingredients remaining by mixing so that the coating is uniform.

3. Cook 1 hour, stirring every 15 minutes.
4. Spread on paper towels to let cool. Store in a tightly closed container.

Nutrition:
Calories 150 Fa 6g Carbs 20g Protein 3g
Sodium 300mg Potassium 93mg
Phosphorus 70mg

Spicy Crab Dip
Preparation Time: 10 minutes
Cooking Time: 20 minutes
Servings: 1
Ingredients:
- 1 can of 8 oz. softened cream cheese
- 1 tbsp. finely chopped onions
- 1 tbsp. lemon juice
- 2 tbsp. Worcestershire sauce
- 1/8 tsp. black pepper Cayenne pepper to taste
- 2 tbsp. to s. of milk or non-fortified rice drink
- 1 can of 6 oz. of crabmeat

Directions:
1. Preheat the oven to 375 degrees F.
2. Pour the cheese cream into a bowl. Add the onions, lemon juice, Worcestershire sauce, black pepper, and cayenne pepper. Mix well. Stir in the milk/rice drink.
3. Add the crabmeat and mix until you obtain a homogeneous mixture.
4. Pour the mixture into a baking dish. Cook without covering for 15 minutes or until bubbles appear. Serve hot with low-sodium crackers or triangle cut pita bread.
5. Microwave until bubbles appear, about 4 minutes, stirring every 1 to 2 minutes.

Nutrition:
Calories 42
Fat 0.5g
Carbs 2g
Protein 7g
Sodium 167mg
Potassium 130mg
Phosphorus 139mg

CHAPTER 10:

Soups and Stews

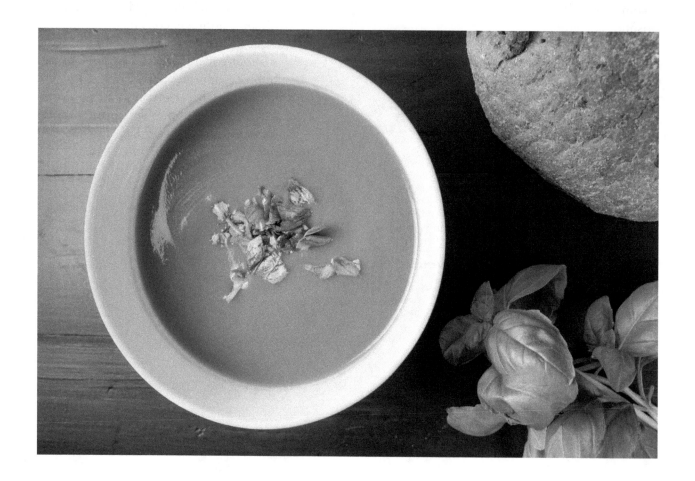

Creamy Tuna Salad

Preparation Time: 10 minutes
Cooking Time: 5 minutes
Servings: 4
Ingredients:

- 3.5 oz. can tuna, drained and flaked
- 1 1/2 tsp garlic powder
- 1 tbsp. dill, chopped
- 1 tsp curry powder
- 2 tbsp. fresh lemon juice
- 1/2 cup onion, chopped
- 1/2 cup celery, chopped
- 1/4 cup parmesan cheese, grated
- 3/4 cup mayonnaise

Directions:

1. Add all ingredients into the large bowl and mix until well combined.
2. Serve and enjoy.

Nutrition:
Calories 224
Fat 15.5g
Carbs 14.1g
Protein 8 g
Phosphorus 110mg
Potassium 117mg
Sodium 75mg

Creamy Mushroom Soup

Preparation Time: 10 minutes
Cooking Time: 15 minutes
Servings: 6
Ingredients:

- 1 lb. mushrooms, sliced
- 1/2 cup heavy cream
- 4 cups chicken broth
- 1 tbsp. sage, chopped
- 1/4 cup butter
- Pepper
- Salt

Directions:

1. Melt butter in a large pot over medium heat.
2. Add sage and sauté for 1 minute.
3. Add mushrooms and cook for 3-5 minutes or until lightly browned.

4. Add broth and stir well and simmer for 5 minutes.
5. Puree the soup using an immersion blender until smooth.
6. Add heavy cream and stir well. Season soup with pepper and salt.
7. Serve hot and enjoy.

Nutrition:
Calories 145
Fat 12.5g
Carbs 3.6g
Protein 5.9g
Phosphorus 140mg
Potassium 127mg
Sodium 75mg

Pork Soup

Preparation Time: 10 minutes
Cooking Time: 4 hours 15 minutes
Servings: 8
Ingredients:

- 2 lbs. country pork ribs, boneless and cut into 1-inch pieces
- 2 cups cauliflower rice
- 1 1/2 tbsp. fresh oregano, chopped
- 1 cup of water
- 2 cups red peppers, chopped
- 1 cup chicken stock
- 1/2 cup dry white wine
- 1 onion, chopped
- 3 garlic cloves, chopped
- 1 tbsp. caper oil
- Pepper
- Salt

Directions:

1. Heat oil in a saucepan over medium heat.
2. Season pork with pepper and salt. Add pork into the saucepan and cook until lightly brown from all the sides.
3. Add onion and garlic and sauté for 2 minutes.
4. Add red peppers, water, stock, and white wine and stir well. Bring to boil.
5. Pour saucepan mixture into the slow cooker.

6. Cover and cook on high for 4 hours.
7. Add cauliflower rice and oregano in the last 20 minutes of cooking.
8. Stir well and serve.

Nutrition:
Calories 263 Fat 15.1g
Carbs 5.8g
Protein 23.4g
Phosphorus 130mg
Potassium 117mg
Sodium 105mg

Thai Chicken Soup
Preparation Time: 10 minutes
Cooking Time: 30 minutes
Servings: 6
Ingredients:

- 4 chicken breasts, slice into 1/4-inch strips
- 1 tbsp. fresh basil, chopped
- 1 tsp ground ginger
- 1 oz. fresh lime juice
- 1 tbsp. coconut aminos
- 2 tbsp. chili garlic paste
- 1/4 cup fish sauce
- 28 oz. water
- 14 oz. chicken broth
- 14 oz. coconut milk

Directions:
1. Add coconut milk, basil, ginger, lime juice, coconut aminos, chili garlic paste, fish sauce, water, and broth into the stockpot. Stir well and bring to boil over medium-high heat.
2. Add chicken and stir well. Turn heat to medium-low and simmer for 30 minutes.
3. Stir well and serve.

Nutrition:
Calories 357
Fat 23.4g
Carbs 5.5g
Protein 31.7g
Phosphorus 110mg
Potassium 117mg
Sodium 75mg

Tasty Pumpkin Soup
Preparation Time: 10 minutes
Cooking Time: 30 minutes
Servings: 6
Ingredients:

- 2 cups pumpkin puree
- 1 cup coconut cream
- 4 cups vegetable broth
- 1/2 tsp ground ginger
- 1 tsp curry powder
- 2 shallots, chopped
- 1/2 onion, chopped
- 4 tbsp. butter
- Pepper
- Salt

Directions:
1. Melt butter in a saucepan over medium heat.
2. Add shallots and onion and sauté until softened.
3. Add ginger and curry powder and stir well.
4. Add broth, pumpkin puree, and coconut cream and stir well. Simmer for 10 minutes.
5. Puree the soup using an immersion blender until smooth.
6. Season with pepper and salt.
7. Serve and enjoy.

Nutrition:
Calories 229 Fat 18.4g
Carbs 13g Protein 5.6g
Phosphorus 120mg Potassium 137mg
Sodium 95mg

Easy Zucchini Soup
Preparation Time: 10 minutes
Cooking Time: 25 minutes
Servings: 4
Ingredients:

- 5 zucchinis, sliced
- 8 oz. cream cheese, softened
- 5 cups vegetable stock
- Pepper
- Salt

Directions:

1. Add zucchini and stock into the stockpot and bring to boil over high heat.
2. Turn heat to medium and simmer for 20 minutes.
3. Add cream cheese and stir until cheese is melted.
4. Puree soup using an immersion blender until smooth.
5. Season with pepper and salt.
6. Serve and enjoy.

Nutrition:

Calories 245
Fat 20.3g
Carbs 10.9g
Protein 7.7g
Phosphorus 110mg
Potassium 117mg
Sodium 75mg

Quick Red pepper Soup

Preparation Time: 10 minutes
Cooking Time: 5 minutes
Servings: 4
Ingredients:

- 28 oz. red pepper, diced
- 1 tbsp. balsamic vinegar
- 1 tbsp. dried basil
- 1 tbsp. dried oregano
- 1 tsp garlic, minced
- 2 tbsp. caper oil
- Pepper
- Salt

Directions:

1. Heat oil in a saucepan over medium heat.
2. Add basil, oregano, and garlic and sauté for 30 seconds.
3. Add red peppers, vinegar, pepper, and salt and simmer for 3 minutes.
4. Stir well and serve hot.

Nutrition:

Calories 108 Fat 7.1g Carbs 11.2g
Protein 2g Phosphorus 130mg
Potassium 127mg Sodium 75mg

Spicy Chicken Soup

Preparation Time: 10 minutes
Cooking Time: 5 minutes
Servings: 4
Ingredients:

- 2 cups cooked chicken, shredded
- 1/2 cup half and half
- 4 cups chicken broth
- 1/3 cup hot sauce
- 3 tbsp. butter
- 4 oz. cream cheese
- Pepper
- Salt

Directions:

1. Add half and half, broth, hot sauce, butter, and cream cheese into the blender and blend until smooth.
2. Pour blended mixture into the saucepan and cook over medium heat until just hot.
3. Add chicken stir well. Season soup with pepper and salt.
4. Serve and enjoy.

Nutrition:

Calories 361 Fat 25.6g
Carbs 3.3g
Protein 28.4g Phosphorus 110mg
Potassium 117mg
Sodium 75mg

Shredded Pork Soup

Preparation Time: 10 minutes
Cooking Time: 8 hours
Servings: 8
Ingredients:

- 1 lb. pork loin
- 8 cups chicken broth
- 2 tsp fresh lime juice
- 1 1/2 tsp garlic powder
- 1 1/2 tsp onion powder
- 1 1/2 tsp chili powder
- 1 1/2 tsp cumin
- 1 jalapeno pepper, minced
- 1 cup onion, chopped
- 3 red peppers, chopped

Directions:

1. Add red peppers, jalapeno, and onion into the slow cooker and stir well.
2. Place meat on top of the red pepper mixture.
3. Pour remaining ingredients on top of the meat.
4. Cover slow cooker and cook on low for 8 hours.
5. Remove meat from slow cooker and shred using a fork.
6. Return shredded meat to the slow cooker and stir well.
7. Serve and enjoy.

Nutrition:
Calories 199
Fat 9.6g
Carbs 6.3g
Protein 21.2g
Phosphorus 140mg
Potassium 127mg
Sodium 95mg

Creamy Chicken Spinach Soup
Preparation Time: 10 minutes
Cooking Time: 10 minutes
Servings: 6
Ingredients:

- 3 cups cooked chicken, shredded
- 1/8 tsp nutmeg
- 4 cup chicken broth
- 1/2 cup parmesan cheese, shredded
- 8 oz. cream cheese
- 1/4 cup butter
- 4 cup baby spinach, chopped
- 1 tsp garlic, minced
- Pepper
- Salt

Directions:

1. Melt butter in a saucepan over medium heat.
2. Add spinach and garlic and cook until spinach is wilted.
3. Add parmesan cheese and cream cheese and stir until cheese is melted.

4. Add remaining ingredients and stir everything well and cook for 5 minutes.
5. Season soup with pepper and salt.
6. Serve and enjoy.

Nutrition:
Calories 361
Fat 25.6g
Carbs 2.8g
Protein 29.5g
Phosphorus 110mg
Potassium 117mg
Sodium 75mg

Creamy Cauliflower Soup
Preparation Time: 10 minutes
Cooking Time: 4 hours
Servings: 5
Ingredients:

- 6 cups cauliflower florets
- 4 oz. mascarpone cheese
- 1 1/2 cup cheddar cheese, shredded
- 1/4 tsp mustard powder
- 3 cups of water
- 1 tsp garlic, minced
- Pepper
- Salt

Directions:

1. Add cauliflower, mustard powder, water, and garlic into the slow cooker and stir well.
2. Cover and cook on low for 4 hours.
3. Stir in cheddar cheese and mascarpone cheese.
4. Puree the soup using an immersion blender until smooth.
5. Season soup with pepper and salt.
6. Serve and enjoy.

Nutrition:
Calories 208
Fat 14.3g
Carbs 7.7g
Protein 13.5g
Phosphorus 210mg
Potassium 157mg
Sodium 85mg

Delicious Curried Chicken Soup

Preparation Time: 10 minutes
Cooking Time: 35 minutes
Servings: 10
Ingredients:

- 5 cups cooked chicken, chopped
- 1/4 cup fresh parsley, chopped
- 1/2 cup sour cream
- 1/4 cup apple cider
- 3 cups celery, chopped
- 1 1/2 tbsp. curry powder
- 10 cups chicken broth
- Pepper
- Salt

Directions:

1. Add all ingredients except sour cream and parsley into the stockpot and stir well.
2. Bring to boil over medium-high heat.
3. Turn heat to medium and simmer for 30 minutes.
4. Add parsley and sour cream and stir well.
5. Season with pepper and salt.
6. Serve and enjoy.

Nutrition:
Calories 180
Fat 6.1g
Carbs 3.7g
Protein 28.9g
Phosphorus 160mg
Potassium 107mg
Sodium 75mg

Delicious Red pepper Basil Soup

Preparation Time: 10 minutes
Cooking Time: 20 minutes
Servings: 6
Ingredients:

- 28 oz. red pepper, diced
- 1 1/2 cups chicken stock
- 1/2 tsp Italian seasoning
- 1/2 tsp garlic, minced
- 1 onion, chopped
- 1/4 cup fresh basil leaves

- 1/2 cup heavy cream
- 2 tbsp. butter
- Pepper
- Salt

Directions:

1. Melt butter in a saucepan over medium-high heat.
2. Add onion and garlic sauté for 5 minutes.
3. Add red peppers, Italian seasoning, and broth. Stir well and bring to boil over high heat.
4. Turn heat to medium-low and simmer for 8-10 minutes.
5. Blend the soup using an immersion blender until smooth.
6. Add heavy cream and basil and stir well. Season soup with pepper and salt.
7. Stir and serve.

Nutrition:
Calories 108
Fat 7.8g
Carbs 9.1g
Protein 1.9g
Phosphorus 110mg
Potassium 137mg
Sodium 95mg

White Fish Stew

Preparation Time: 10 minutes
Cooking Time: 35 minutes
Servings: 3
Ingredients:

- 4 white fish fillets
- 1 cup of water
- 1 onion, sliced
- 1/2 tsp paprika
- 1/4 cup caper oil
- 1/4 tsp pepper
- 1 tsp salt

Directions:

1. Add caper oil, paprika, onion, water, pepper, and salt into the saucepan. Stir well and bring to boil over medium-high heat.

2. Turn heat to medium-low and simmer for 15 minutes.
3. Add white fish fillets and cook until fish is cooked.
4. Serve and enjoy.

Nutrition:
Calories 513
Fat 32.3g
Carbs 3.7g
Protein 50.7g
Phosphorus 120mg
Potassium 117mg
Sodium 75mg

Carrot Cauliflower Soup
Preparation Time: 10 minutes
Cooking Time: 25 minutes
Servings: 8
Ingredients:
- 4 carrots, shredded
- 1 cauliflower head, chopped
- 8 cups chicken broth
- 1 onion, diced
- 5 oz. coconut milk
- 1 tbsp. caper oil
- 1 tbsp. curry powder
- 1/2 tsp turmeric powder
- 1/2 tbsp. ginger, grated
- Pepper
- Salt

Directions:
1. Heat oil in a saucepan over medium heat.
2. Add onion and sauté for 5 minutes.
3. Add cauliflower, carrots, and broth and bring to boil.
4. Turn heat to medium-low and simmer until veggie is softened.
5. Add curry powder, turmeric, and ginger and stir well.
6. Blend the soup using a blender until smooth.
7. Add coconut milk and stir well.
8. Season soup with pepper and salt.
9. Serve and enjoy.

Nutrition:
Calories 125
Fat 7.5g
Carbs 8.7g
Protein 6.5g
Phosphorus 210mg
Potassium 187mg
Sodium 105mg

Pumpkin, Coconut and Sage Soup
Preparation Time: 10 minutes
Cooking Time: 30 minutes
Servings: 3
Ingredients:
- 1 cup pumpkin, canned
- 6 cups chicken broth
- 1 cup low fat coconut almond milk
- 1 teaspoon sage, chopped
- 3 garlic cloves, peeled
- Sunflower seeds and pepper to taste

Directions:
1. Take a stockpot and add all the ingredients except coconut almond milk into it.
2. Place stockpot over medium heat.
3. Let it bring to a boil.
4. Reduce heat to simmer for 30 minutes.
5. Add the coconut almond milk and stir.
6. Serve bacon and enjoy!

Nutrition:
Calories 145
Fat 12g
Carbs 8g
Protein 6g
Phosphorus 110mg
Potassium 117mg
Sodium 75mg

Sweet Squash and Leek Soup
Preparation Time: 10 minutes
Cooking Time: 8 hours
Servings: 6
Ingredients:
- 6 cups sweet squash, peeled and cubed

- 2 leeks, whites and greens, sliced
- 6 cups vegetable stock
- 1 teaspoon dried thyme
- 1 teaspoon salt
- ¼ teaspoon fresh ground black pepper

Directions:

1. Add sweet squash, leeks, thyme, stock, salt and pepper to your Slow Cooker.
2. Close lid and cook on LOW for 8 hours.
3. Mash with potato masher/ use an immersion blender to smooth the soup.
4. Serve and enjoy!

Nutrition:

Calories 234
Fat 2g
Carbs 47g
Protein 8g
Phosphorus 120mg
Potassium 137mg
Sodium 75mg

Japanese Onion Soup

Preparation Time: 15 minutes
Cooking Time: 45 minutes
Servings: 4
Ingredients:

- ½ stalk celery, diced
- 1 small onion, diced
- ½ carrot, diced
- 1 teaspoon fresh ginger root, grated
- ¼ teaspoon fresh garlic, minced
- 2 tablespoons chicken stock
- 3 teaspoons beef bouillon granules
- 1 cup fresh shiitake, mushrooms
- 2 quarts water
- 1 cup baby Portobello mushrooms, sliced
- 1 tablespoon fresh chives

Directions:

1. Take a saucepan and place it over high heat, add water, bring to a boil.
2. Add beef bouillon, celery, onion, chicken stock, and carrots, half of the mushrooms, ginger, and garlic.

3. Put on the lid and reduce heat to medium, cook for 45 minutes.
4. Take another saucepan and add another half of mushrooms.
5. Once the soup is cooked, strain the soup into the pot with uncooked mushrooms.
6. Garnish with chives and enjoy!

Nutrition:

Calories 25 Fat 0.2g
Carbs 5g Protein 1.4g Phosphorus 210mg
Potassium 217mg Sodium 75mg

Amazing Broccoli and Cauliflower Soup

Preparation Time: 10 minutes
Cooking Time: 8 hours
Servings: 4
Ingredients:

- 3 cups broccoli florets
- 2 cups cauliflower florets
- 2 garlic cloves, minced
- ½ cup shallots, chopped
- 1 carrot, chopped
- 3 ½ cups low sodium veggie stick
- Pinch of pepper
- 1 cup fat-free milk
- 6 ounces low-fat cheddar, shredded
- 1 cup non-fat Greek yogurt

Directions:

1. Add broccoli, cauliflower, garlic, shallots, carrot, stock, and pepper to your Slow Cooker.
2. Stir well and place lid.
3. Cook on LOW for 8 hours.
4. Add milk and cheese.
5. Use an immersion blender to smooth the soup.
6. Add yogurt and blend once more.
7. Ladle into bowls and enjoy!

Nutrition:

Calories 218 Fat 11g
Carbs 15g Protein 12g
Phosphorus 206mg
Potassium 147mg Sodium 75mg

Pumpkin and Walnut Puree

Preparation Time: 10 minutes
Cooking Time: 10 minutes
Servings: 6
Ingredients:

- 100 g walnuts, without shell
- 300 g pumpkin
- 30 ml of milk
- 600 ml of water

Directions:

1. Peel the walnuts and pound them with the mortar.
2. Peel the pumpkin and cut into pieces. Place the pumpkin pieces in a plastic bag and place it in the microwave over a high temperature for five minutes.
3. Put the water with the pumpkin and walnuts in the blender and puree.
4. Put everything in a saucepan and cook until mushy over low heat.
5. Slowly pour in the milk and stir.

Nutrition:
Calories 53
Protein 2g
Carbs 4g
Fat 4g
Sodium 167mg
Potassium 201mg
Phosphorus 59mg
Fiber 1.2g

Bean and Pepper Soup with Coriander

Preparation Time: 30 minutes
Cooking Time: 20 minutes
Servings: 4
Ingredients:

- 1 onion
- 2 garlic cloves
- 2 tbsp. caper oil
- 2 red peppers
- 800 ml vegetable broth
- salt
- cayenne pepper
- Tabasco
- curry powder
- 2 cans kidney beans á 240 g
- 200 ml whipped cream at least 30% fat content
- 1 coriander

Directions:

1. Peel the onion and garlic, diced finely, and sauté in a saucepan with hot oil until translucent. Wash the bell peppers, cut in half, core, dice, and add. Sweat briefly and deglaze with the broth. Season with salt, cayenne pepper, curry, and Tabasco and simmer over medium heat for 10 minutes.
2. Pour the beans over a sieve, rinse with cold water and drain well.
3. Stir the cream with the beans into the soup and simmer for another 4 minutes.
4. Wash the coriander, shake dry, pluck the leaves off, and roughly chop.
5. Season the soup to taste, season again if necessary, pour into preheated bowls, and serve sprinkled with the coriander. Serve with a fresh baguette if you like.

Nutrition:
Calories 357
Protein 14g
Phosphorus: 112mg
Potassium 132mg
Sodium 222 mg
Fat 22 g
Carbs 26g

Bean and Ham Soup with Bread

Preparation Time: 30 minutes
Cooking Time: 1h
Servings: 4
Ingredients:

- 1 onion
- 2 garlic cloves
- 250 g sweet squash
- 1 red chili pepper
- 100 g ham
- 2 tbsp. vegetable oil

- 1 l meat soup
- 100 g dried kidney beans
- 100 g dried white lima bean
- 250 g pizza red peppers
- 2 tbsp. red pepper paste
- Tabasco
- Salt
- Pepper from the mill
- 4 rye rolls

Directions:
1. Mix the beans, pour water over them, and leave to soak overnight. The next day, peel and finely chop the onion and garlic. Wash the chili pepper, slit lengthways, core, and chop very finely. Finely dice the ham. Peel the sweet potato and cut into pieces of equal size.
2. Heat the oil in a large saucepan, sauté the onions and garlic until translucent. Fry the ham and red pepper paste in it, season with salt and pepper. Add the chili and sweet squash and fry briefly. Add the stock and beans (without soaking water), mash the red peppers with a fork, and add to the beans.
3. Season with Tabasco and cover and simmer over low heat for about 30-40 minutes. If necessary, add some more broth and season the bean soup to taste. Serve with the rye rolls.

Nutrition:
Calories 181 Carbs 33.5g
Protein 10.3g
Fibers 9.3g
Sodium 0.5g
Phosphorous 31.9mg
Potassium 387.1mg

Hearty Vegetable Soup with Bacon
Preparation Time 12h
Cooking Time: 1 h 15 minutes
Servings: 4
Ingredients:

- 250 g dried kidney beans

- 150 g smoked bacon
- 1 large onion
- 2 garlic cloves
- 3 red peppers
- 1 small savoy cabbage
- 4 squash
- 2 tbsp. caper oil
- 1 ½ l meat soup
- salt
- pepper from the mill

Directions:
1. Soak the beans with cold water and leave overnight.
2. Drain the beans and cook them halfway through in fresh cold water for about 30–40 minutes.
3. In the meantime, dice the bacon. Peel onion and garlic and chop finely. Scald the red peppers with boiling water for a few seconds, rinse, peel, quarter, core, and chop.
4. Clean and wash the cabbage, quarter lengthways, cut off the stalk, and cut the quarters crosswise into strips. Peel the squash and cut into bite-sized pieces.
5. A sauce pan heats the caper oil and briefly brown the onions, garlic cloves, and bacon. Pour the meat stock. Add red peppers, savoy cabbage strips, and squash. Drain the beans and stir into the stock under the vegetables. Salt and pepper and let simmer on low heat for about 30 minutes.

Nutrition:
Calories 567
Protein 17g
Phosphorus: 112mg
Potassium 132mg
Sodium 222mg
Fat 40g
Carbs 36g

Mexican-Style Chicken and Vegetable Soup

Preparation Time: 40 minutes
Cooking Time: 2 h 10 minutes
Servings: 4
Ingredients:

- 1 soup chicken
- 3 onions
- 2 carrots
- 150 g celery root
- 1 bay leaf
- 2 cloves
- 1 tsp peppercorns
- 1 tbsp. rapeseed oil
- 2 green peppers
- 1 red chili pepper
- 6 red peppers
- 1 can of kidney beans
- 1 can corn
- salt
- pepper

Directions:

1. Wash the chicken soup and cover it with cold water in a saucepan that is large enough. Simmer. Boil. Meanwhile, peel 2 onions, carrots, and celery, and roughly dice them.
2. Add the bay leaves, cloves, and peppercorns to the chicken and cook for about 2 hours, over medium heat. If necessary, skim off the foam occasionally and add water.
3. Take the chicken out of the soup. Strain the stock and measure 1 liter (otherwise use the remainder). Peel the chicken and the skin is removed. Have the meat cut into strips.
4. Peel the remaining onion and dice it. In a saucepan, sweat in hot oil until it is translucent. Pour the stock into it and bring it to a boil. In the meantime, wash, cut in half, clean and dice the peppers and chili. Scald the hot-water red peppers, rinse, peel, quarter, core, and dice. Drain

the beans and maize and add bell pepper, chili, red peppers, and chicken to the soup.

5. For about 15 minutes, let everything simmer together. Season with pepper and salt and serve.

Nutrition:
Calories 69
Protein 5.13g
Carbs 7.87g
Fat 2.01g
Sodium 347 mg
Potassium 153mg
Phosphorous 44mg

Mexican Bean Soup

Preparation Time: 20 minutes
Cooking Time: 25 minutes
Servings: 4
Ingredients:

- 4 red peppers
- 150 g green beans
- 1 onion
- 1 clove of garlic
- 1 red chili pepper
- 2 tbsp. caper oil
- 2 tbsp. red pepper paste
- 1 tsp paprika noble sweet
- 1 tsp ground cumin
- 1 tsp ground coriander
- 1 l vegetable broth
- 240 g kidney beans (can; drained weight)
- 240 g white beans (can; drained weight)
- Salt
- Pepper
- Coriander greens for garnish

Directions:

1. Scald, quench, peel, remove the stalk and roughly chop the red peppers with hot water. Wash the green beans, clean them, and cut them into small pieces.

2. Wash and clean the chili, remove the seeds and, if desired, finely chop it.

3. Sauté onion garlic and chilly. Sauté the red pepper paste and add paprika, cumin, and cilantro to the mixture. Put the broth in and bring it to a boil. Add the green beans and red peppers and simmer over low heat for about 10 minutes. The kidney and white beans are drained, washed, and added.

4. Let it simmer more for 5 minutes. Serve in bowls with coriander leaves and season with salt and pepper.

Nutrition:
Calories 205
Phosphorus 112mg
Potassium 132mg
Sodium 222mg
Protein 13g
Fat 6g
Carbs 23g

Clear Soup with Vegetables
Preparation Time: 20 minutes
Cooking Time: 20 minutes
Serving: 4
Ingredients:

- 200 g waxy squash
- 2 poles celery
- 4 spring onions
- 1 onion
- 2 garlic cloves
- 2 yellow peppers
- 2 tbsp. caper oil
- 1 tbsp. red pepper paste
- 1 l vegetable broth
- 400 g kidney beans can
- 2 fresh bay leaves
- salt
- pepper

Directions:

1. Peel and dice the squash, clean and wash the celery and spring onions and cut into rings. Peel and chop the onion and garlic. Clean the peppers,

cut in half, remove the seeds and white skins, wash and cut into thin strips.

2. Heat the oil in a hot saucepan and sauté the vegetables for 2-3 minutes over medium heat.

3. Fry the red pepper paste briefly, then pour in the stock and bring to the boil once. In the meantime, drain the beans and wash them.

4. Add to the clear soup together with the bay leaf.

5. Season

6. Simmer over low heat for about 15 minutes.

7. Season the soup again to taste and serve in bowls.

Nutrition:
Calories 227 Protein 12g
Fat 6g Phosphorus 112mg
Potassium 132mg Sodium 222 mg
Carbs 30g

Bean Stew with Beef Fillet
Preparation Time: 20 minutes
Cooking Time: 25 minutes
Servings: 4
Ingredients:

- 50 g kidney beans (can; drained weight)
- 50 g small white beans (can; drained weight)
- ½ onion
- 1 small clove of garlic
- ½ red pepper
- 2 tsp caper oil
- 1 branch thyme
- 1 bay leaf
- 200 chunky red peppers (can)
- salt
- pepper
- cayenne pepper
- ¼ tsp ground coriander
- 150 g beef fillet
- 1 stem basil

Directions:

1. In a sieve, rinse both types of beans and let them drain. Peel the garlic and onion and cut them into fine cubes. Wash, clean, core, and slice the peppers.
2. In a casserole, heat one teaspoon of oil. Sauté the onion and garlic in it over medium heat for 2 minutes. Wash the thyme and the bay leaves and add the beans and red peppers to the saucepan, season with salt, pepper, cayenne pepper, and coriander and cook for about 15-17 minutes over medium heat, stirring occasionally.
3. Cut the beef into thin strips about 20 minutes before cooking time ends. In a pan, heat the remaining oil. For 2-3 minutes, fry the beef fillet strips over high heat. With salt and pepper, season.
4. Wash the basil, shake it dry, and finely chop it. Top the bean stew with the meat and basil.

Nutrition:

Calories 393
Protein 40g
Phosphorus 112mg
Potassium 132mg
Sodium 222mg
Fat 17g
Carbs 19g

Nutmeg Pumpkin Soup with Kidney Beans

Preparation Time: 20 minutes
Cooking Time: 20 minutes
Servings: 4
Ingredients:

- 1 kg nutmeg pumpkin
- 2 dice vegetable broth
- 1 tbsp. caper oil
- 1 lemon
- 400 g kidney beans (1 can, drained weight)
- 2 stems parsley
- pepper
- salt

Directions:

1. The pumpkin is cleaned and peeled, the core removed and the pulp cut into cubes. In a saucepan, put the pumpkin cubes in. Add sufficient water just to cover the pumpkin.
2. When boiling add 2 cubes of stock. Cook for 20 minutes over medium heat until the pumpkin is tender.
3. Squeeze the juice of the lemon.
4. In a colander drain the kidney beans and rinse with hot water.
5. Wash the parsley, shake it dry and, except for a few leaves, chop finely.
6. Add the oil to the pumpkin at the end of the cooking time and finely puree it with a hand blender. Season with lemon juice, pepper, and a little salt if necessary. Distribute the beans and pour hot soup over them on 4 soup plates. Serve with parsley, sprinkled.

Nutrition:

Calories 197
Protein 12 g
Fat 4 g
Phosphorus 112mg
Potassium 132mg
Sodium 222mg
Carbs 27g

Zucchini Soup

Preparation Time: 20 minutes
Cooking Time: 20 minutes
Servings: 4
Ingredients:

- 2 large zucchinis
- 1 onion
- 2 squash
- 2 carrots
- 1 tbsp. (sesame oil, coconut fat, refined rapeseed or caper oil) frying oil
- 500 ml vegetable broth

- 100 g (natural, 15% fat in dry matter) cream cheese
- ½ bunch of parsley
- Salt and pepper

Directions:

1. Wash and dice the zucchini. Peel the onion, squash, and carrots, then dice them.
2. Heat the oil in a pot. Sweat the onion cubes in it until they are golden yellow. Add the rest of the vegetables and fry briefly.
3. Deglaze with the vegetable stock
4. Simmer for about 10 minutes.
5. Puree the soup.
6. Stir the cream cheese into the warm soup and season with salt and pepper. Wash and finely chop the parsley and serve on top of the soup.

Nutrition:
Calories 36.04
Carbs 4.07g
Phosphorus: 112mg
Potassium 132mg
Sodium 222mg
Protein 2.38g

Quick Pea Soup

Preparation Time: 5 minutes
Cooking Time: 15 minutes
Servings: 3
Ingredients:

- 300 g Squash
- 1 onion
- 1 toe garlic
- 30 g butter
- 200 g cream
- 1 Bay leaf
- 400 g frozen peas
- Salt
- Pepper
- Nutmeg
- Cumin
- As required: smoked salmon

Directions:

1. Peel the squash, onion, and garlic and cut into cubes.
2. Melt the butter and sauté squash, onions, and garlic in it.
3. Deglaze with cream, fill the cup twice with water and add this as well. Season with salt, pepper, freshly grated nutmeg, and cumin.
4. Add the bay leaf and cook everything until the squash are done. Take out the bay leaf and add the peas.
5. Bring to the boil again and then puree with a hand blender. If the soup is still too thick, add 1 more shot of water.
6. Season again to taste and serve. Add smoked salmon strips to the soup to taste.

Nutrition:
Calories 61
Protein 3.2g
Carbs 9.88g
Calcium 12mg
Phosphorous 47mg
Potassium 71mg
Sodium 336mg

Red pepper Soup Made from Fresh Red peppers

Preparation Time: 20 minutes
Cooking Time: 20 minutes
Servings: 2
Ingredients:

- 1 kg of red peppers
- 200 ml of water
- ½ teaspoon salt
- 1 sprig of rosemary
- 1 sprig of thyme
- 2 tbsp. cream
- 2 tbsp. sour cream

Directions:

1. Wash the red peppers and put them in a saucepan with water and salt. Bring to a boil. Simmer for until the

peel starts to peel off the red peppers and the red peppers are soft.

2. In the meantime, wash the herbs and let them dry on kitchen paper.

3. Drain the red peppers, collecting the cooking water if necessary. Strain or strain the soft red peppers through a sieve. Let the pureed red peppers simmer for about 10 minutes. Then stir with the cream until smooth. Dilute with some of the collected cooking water as desired.

4. Strip off the rosemary and thyme needles and chop finely. Pour the soup into two bowls, put a dollop of sour cream on top and sprinkle everything with the herbs.

Nutrition:
Calories186
Protein 6g
Fat 8g
Phosphorus: 112mg
Potassium 132mg
Sodium 222 mg
Carbs 21g

Chickpea Soup with Croutons

Preparation Time: 20 minutes
Cooking Time: 45 minutes
Servings: 1 – 4
Ingredients:

- Dried chickpeas 60 g
- Common bread without salt 80 g
- Extra virgin caper oil 20 g
- Rosemary
- Sage
- Garlic
- Bay leaf
- Chili

Directions:

1. Soak the chickpeas the night before.
2. Bring to a boil to pots of water.
3. Meanwhile, prepare a sauté with chopped rosemary, a bit of garlic, oil, sage, a few bay leaves, and a little

chili. When the garlic is golden, it should be removed.

4. Pour the chickpeas into boiling water, drain them after a quarter of an hour and dip them back into the second pot of boiling water. Leave to cook for another quarter of an hour.

5. Add some chickpeas to the mixture and place them in a small pan with some of their water. The others must be blended to create a cream that we can make more or less thick with your water. Add the whole chickpeas, bring to the boil again and add the common pasta.

6. Serve accompanied with common wood baked toasted bread, adding a drizzle of extra virgin caper oil.

Nutrition:
Calories 594
Protein 23g
Phosphorous 241mg
Potassium 609 mg
Carbs 81g
Sodium 8mg

Chicken Wild Rice Soup

Preparation Time: 10 minutes
Cooking Time: 15 minutes
Servings: 6
Ingredients:

- 2/3 cup wild rice, uncooked
- 1 tbsp. onion, chopped finely
- 1 tbsp. fresh parsley, chopped
- 1 cup carrots, chopped
- 8 oz. chicken breast, cooked
- 2 tbsp. butter
- 1/4 cup all-purpose white flour
- 5 cups low-sodium chicken broth
- 1 tbsp. slivered almonds

Directions:

1. Start by adding rice and 2 cups broth along with ½ cup water to a cooking pot.
2. Cook until the rice soft and set it aside.

3. Melt butter in a saucepan.
4. Stir in onion and sauté until soft then add the flour and the remaining broth.
5. Cook while stirring for 1 minute then add the chicken, cooked rice, and carrots.
6. Cook for 5 minutes on simmer.
7. Garnish with almonds.
8. Serve fresh.

Nutrition:
Calories 287
Protein 21g
Carbs 35g
Fat 7g
Sodium 182mg
Potassium 384mg
Phosphorus 217mg
Fiber 1.6g

Chicken Noodle Soup
Preparation Time: 10 minutes
Cooking Time: 25 minutes
Servings: 2
Ingredients:
- 1 1/2 cups low-sodium vegetable broth
- 1 cup of water
- 1/4 tsp poultry seasoning
- 1/4 tsp black pepper
- 1 cup chicken strips
- 1/4 cup carrot
- 2 oz. egg noodles, uncooked

Directions:
1. Cook soup on high heat for 25 minutes in a slow cooker.
2. Serve warm.

Nutrition:
Calories 103
Protein 8g
Carbs 11g
Fat 3g
Sodium 355mg
Potassium 264mg
Phosphorus 128mg
Fiber 4g

CHAPTER 11:

Vegetables

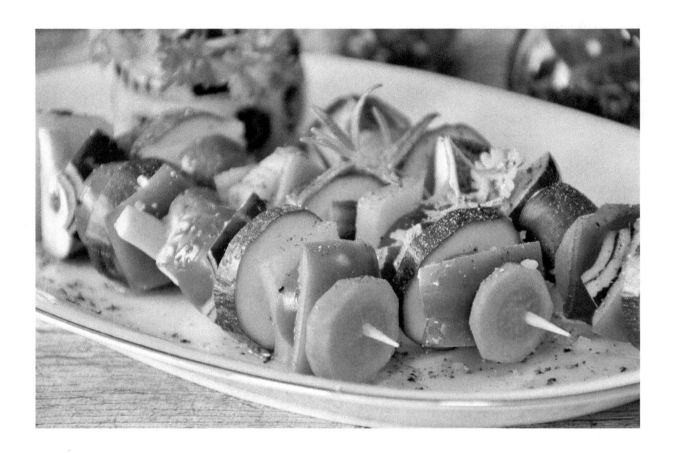

Sautéed Green Beans

Preparation Time: 10 minutes
Cooking Time: 15 minutes
Servings: 4
Ingredients:

- 2 cup frozen green beans
- ½ cup red bell pepper
- 4 tsp margarine
- ¼ cup onion
- 1 tsp dried dill weed
- 1 tsp dried parsley
- ¼ tsp black pepper

Directions:

1. Cook green beans in a large pan of boiling water until tender, then drain.
2. 2. While the beans are cooking, melt the margarine in a skillet and fry the other vegetables.
3. Add the beans to sautéed vegetables.
4. Sprinkle with freshly ground pepper and serve with meat and fish dishes.

Nutrition:
Calories 67
Carbs 8g
Protein 4g
Sodium 5mg
Potassium 179mg
Phosphorous 32mg

Garlicky Penne Pasta with Asparagus

Preparation Time: 10 minutes
Cooking Time: 10 minutes
Servings: 4
Ingredients:

- 2 tbsp. butter
- 1lb asparagus, cut into 2-inch pieces
- 2 tsp lemon juice
- 4 cup whole wheat penne pasta, cooked
- ¼ cup shredded Parmesan cheese
- ¼ tsp Tabasco® hot sauce

Directions:

1. Add caper oil and butter in a skillet over medium heat.
2. Fry garlic and red pepper flakes for 2-3 minutes.

3. Add asparagus, Tabasco sauce, lemon juice, and black pepper to skillet and cook for a further 6 minutes.
4. Add hot pasta and cheese. Toss and serve.

Nutrition:
Calories 387
Carbs 49g
Protein 13g
Sodium 93mg
Potassium 258mg
Phosphorous 252mg

Garlic Mashed Squash

Preparation Time: 5 minutes
Cooking Time: 20 minutes
Servings: 4
Ingredients:

- 2 medium squash, peeled and sliced
- ¼ cup butter
- ¼ cup 1% low-fat milk
- 2 garlic cloves

Directions:

1. Double-boil or soak the squash to reduce potassium if you are on a low potassium diet.
2. Boil squash and garlic until soft. Drain.
3. Beat the squash and garlic with butter and milk until smooth.

Nutrition:
Calories 168
Carbs 29g
Protein 5g
Sodium 59
Potassium 161g
Phosphorous 57mg

Ginger Glazed Carrots

Preparation Time: 10 minutes
Cooking Time: 20 minutes
Servings: 4
Ingredients:

- 2 cups carrots, sliced into 1-inch pieces
- ¼ cup apple juice
- 2 tbsp. margarine, melted
- ¼ cup boiling water
- 1 tbsp. sugar

- 1 tsp cornstarch
- ¼ tsp salt
- ¼ tsp ground ginger

Directions:

1. Cook carrots until tender.
2. Mix sugar, cornstarch, salt, ginger, apple juice, and margarine together
3. Pour mixture over carrots and cook for 10 minutes until thickened.

Nutrition:

Calories 101
Fat 3g
Carbs 14g
Protein 1g
Sodium 87
Potassium 202g
Phosphorous 26mg

Carrot-Apple Casserole

Preparation Time: 15 minutes
Cooking Time: 50 minutes
Servings: 8
Ingredients:

- 6 large carrots, peeled and sliced
- 4 large apples, peeled and sliced
- 3 tbsp. butter
- ½ cup apple juice
- 5 tbsp. all-purpose flour
- 2 tbsp. brown sugar
- ½ tsp ground nutmeg

Directions:

1. Preheat oven to 350° F.
2. Let the carrots boil for 5 minutes or until tender. Drain.
3. Arrange the carrots and apples in a large casserole dish.
4. Mix the flour, brown sugar, and nutmeg in a small bowl.
5. Rub in butter to make a crumb topping.
6. Sprinkle the crumb over the carrots and apples, then drizzle with juice.
7. Bake until bubbling and golden brown.

Nutrition:

Calories 245 Fat 6g Carbs 49g
Protein 1g Sodium 91mg
Potassium 169mg Phosphorous 17mg

Creamy Shells with Peas and Bacon

Preparation Time: 15 minutes
Cooking Time: 15 minutes
Servings: 4
Ingredients:

- 1 cup part-skim ricotta cheese
- ½ cup grated Parmesan cheese
- 3 slices bacon, cut into strips
- 1 cup onion, chopped
- ¾ cup of frozen green peas
- 1 tbsp. caper oil
- ¼ tsp black pepper
- 3 garlic cloves, minced
- 3 cup cooked whole-wheat small shell pasta
- 1 tbsp. lemon juice
- 2 tbsp. unsalted butter

Directions:

1. Place ricotta, Parmesan cheese, butter, and pepper in a large bowl.
2. Cook bacon in a skillet until crisp. Set aside.
3. Add the garlic and onion to the same skillet and fry until soft. Add to bowl with ricotta.
4. Cook the peas and add to the ricotta.
5. Add half a cup of the reserved cooking water and lemon juice to the ricotta mixture and mix well.
6. Add the pasta, bacon, and peas to the bowl and mix well.
7. Put freshly ground black pepper and serve.

Nutrition:

Calories 429
Fat 14g
Carbs 27g
Protein 13g
Sodium 244mg
Potassium 172mg
Phosphorous 203mg

Double-Boiled Stewed Squash

Preparation Time: 20 minutes
Cooking Time: 30 minutes
Servings: 4
Ingredients:

- 2 cup squash, diced into ½ inch cubes
- ½ cup hot water
- ½ cup liquid non-dairy creamer
- ¼ tsp garlic powder
- ¼ tsp black pepper
- 2 tbsp. margarine
- 2 tsp all-purpose white flour

Directions:

1. Soak or double boil the squash if you are on a low potassium diet.
2. Boil squash for 15 minutes.
3. Drain squash and return to pan. Add half a cup of hot water, the creamer, garlic powder, pepper, and margarine. Heat to a boil.
4. Mix the flour with a tablespoon of water and then stir this into the squash. Cook for 3 minutes until the mixture has thickened and the flour has cooked.

Nutrition:
Calories 184
Carbs 25g
Protein 2g
Potassium 161mg
Phosphorous 65mg
Sodium 3mg

Double-Boiled Country Style Fried Squash

Preparation Time: 20 minutes
Cooking Time: 20 minutes
Servings: 4
Ingredients:

- 2 medium squash, cut into large chips
- ½ cup canola oil
- ¼ tsp ground cumin
- ¼ tsp paprika
- ¼ tsp white pepper
- 3 tbsp. ketchup

Directions:

1. Soak or double boil the squash if you are on a low potassium diet.
2. Heat oil over medium heat in a skillet.
3. Fry the squash for around 10 minutes until golden brown.
4. Drain squash, then sprinkle with cumin, pepper, and paprika.
5. Serve with ketchup or mayo.

Nutrition:
Calories 156 Fat 0.1g
Carbs 21g
Protein 2g
Sodium 3mg
Potassium 296mg
Phosphorous 34mg

Broccoli-Onion Latkes

Preparation Time: 15 minutes
Cooking Time: 20 minutes
Servings: 4
Ingredients:

- 3 cups broccoli florets, diced
- ½ cup onion, chopped
- 2 large eggs, beaten
- 2 tbsp. all-purpose white flour
- 2 tbsp. caper oil

Directions:

1. Cook the broccoli for around 5 minutes until tender. Drain.
2. Mix the flour into the eggs.
3. Combine the onion, broccoli, and egg mixture and stir through.
4. Prepare caper oil in a skillet on medium-high heat.
5. Drop a spoon of the mixture onto the pan to make 4 latkes.
6. Cook each side until golden brown.
7. Drain on a paper towel and serve.

Nutrition:
Calories 140
Fat 10g
Carbs 7g
Protein 6g
Sodium 58mg
Potassium 276mg
Phosphorous 101mg

Cranberry Cabbage

Preparation Time: 10 minutes
Cooking Time: 20 minutes
Servings: 8
Ingredients:

- 10 ounces canned whole-berry cranberry sauce
- 1 tablespoon fresh lemon juice
- 1 medium head red cabbage
- 1/4 teaspoon ground cloves

Directions:

1. Place the cranberry sauce, lemon juice, and cloves in a large pan and bring to the boil.
2. Add the cabbage and reduce it to a simmer.
3. Cook until the cabbage is tender, occasionally stirring to make sure the sauce does not stick.
4. Delicious served with beef, lamb, or pork.

Nutrition:
Calories 73
Fat 0g
Carbs 18g
Protein 1g
Sodium 32mg
Potassium 138mg
Phosphorous 18mg

Cauliflower Rice

Preparation Time: 5 minutes
Cooking Time: 10 minutes
Servings: 1
Ingredients:

- 1 small head cauliflower cut into florets
- 1 tbsp. butter
- ¼ tsp black pepper
- ¼ tsp garlic powder
- ¼ tsp salt-free herb seasoning blend

Directions:

1. Blitz cauliflower pieces in a food processor until it has a grain-like consistency.
2. Melt butter in a saucepan and add spices.
3. Add the cauliflower rice grains and cook over low-medium heat for approximately 10 minutes.
4. Use a fork to fluff the rice before serving.
5. Serve as an alternative to rice with curries, stews, and starch to accompany meat and fish dishes.

Nutrition:
Calories 47
Fat 12g
Carbs 4g
Protein 1g
Sodium 300mg
Potassium 206mg
Phosphorous 31mg

CHAPTER 12:

Salads

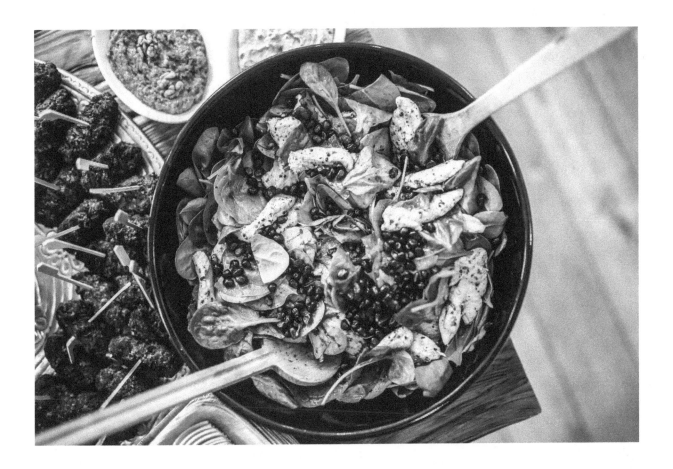

Pear & Brie Salad
Preparation Time: 5 minutes
Cooking Time: 0 minutes
Servings: 4
Ingredients:

- 1 tablespoon caper oil
- 1 cup arugula
- ½ lemon
- ½ cup canned pears
- ¼ cucumber
- ¼ cup chopped brie

Directions:

1. Peel and dice the cucumber.
2. Dice the pear.
3. Wash the arugula.
4. Combine salad in a serving bowl and crumble the brie over the top.
5. Whisk the caper oil and lemon juice together.
6. Drizzle over the salad.
7. Season with a little black pepper to taste and serve immediately.

Nutrition :
Calories 54
Protein 1 g
Carbs 12 g
Fat 7 g
Sodium 57mg
Potassium 115 mg
Phosphorus 67 mg

Caesar Salad
Preparation Time: 5 minutes
Cooking Time: 5 minutes
Servings: 4
Ingredients:

- 1 head romaine lettuce
- ¼ cup mayonnaise
- 1 tablespoon lemon juice
- anchovy fillets
- 1 teaspoon Worcestershire sauce
- Black pepper
- garlic cloves
- tablespoons. Parmesan cheese
- 1 teaspoon mustard

Directions:

1. In a bowl mix all ingredients and mix well
2. Serve with dressing

Nutrition:
Calories 44
Fat 2.1 g
Carbs 4.3g
Protein 3.2g
Phosphorus 45.6mg
Potassium 27mg
Sodium 121 mg

Thai Cucumber Salad
Preparation Time: 5 minutes
Cooking Time: 5 minutes
Servings: 2
Ingredients:

- ¼ cup chopped peanuts
- ¼ cup white sugar
- ½ cup cilantro
- ¼ cup rice wine vinegar
- cucumbers
- 2 jalapeno peppers

Directions:

1. Add all ingredients in a small basin and combine well
2. Serve with dressing

Nutrition:
Calories 20
Fat 0g
Sodium 85mg
Carbs 5g
Protein 1g
Potassium 190.4mg
Phosphorus 46.8mg

Barb's Asian Slaw
Preparation Time: 5 minutes
Cooking Time: 5 minutes
Servings: 2
Ingredients:

- 1 cabbage head, shredded
- chopped green onions
- ½ cup slivered or sliced almonds

Dressing:

- ½ cup caper oil
- ¼ cup tamari or soy sauce
- 1 tablespoon honey or maple syrup
- 1 tablespoon baking stevia

Directions:

1 Heat up dressing ingredients in a saucepan on the stove until thoroughly mixed.
2 Mix all ingredients when you are ready to serve.

Nutrition :

Calories 205 Protein 27g
Carbs 12g Fat 10g Phosphorous 76mg
Potassium 27mg
Sodium 111mg

Green Bean and Potato Salad

Preparation Time: 5 minutes
Cooking Time: 5 minutes
Servings: 4
Ingredients:

- ½ cup basil
- ¼ cup caper oil
- 1 tablespoon mustard
- ¾ lb. green beans
- 1 tablespoon lemon juice
- ½ cup balsamic vinegar
- 1 red onion
- 1 lb. red squash
- 1 garlic clove

Directions:

1 Place squash in a pot with water and bring to a boil for 15-18 minutes or until tender
2 Thrown in green beans after 5-6 minutes
3 Drain and cut into cubes
4 In a bowl add all ingredients and mix well
5 Serve with dressing

Nutrition:

Calories 153.2 Fat 2.0 g
Sodium 77.6 mg Potassium 759mg
Carbs 29g Protein 6.9g
Phosphorus 49mg

Italian Cucumber Salad

Preparation Time: 5 minutes
Cooking Time: 0 minutes
Servings: 2
Ingredients:

- 1/4 cup rice vinegar
- 1/8 teaspoon stevia
- 1/2 teaspoon caper oil
- 1/8 teaspoon black pepper
- 1/2 cucumber, sliced
- 1 cup carrots, sliced
- tablespoons green onion, sliced
- tablespoons red bell pepper, sliced
- 1/2 teaspoon Italian seasoning blend

Directions:

1 Put all the salad ingredients into a suitable salad bowl.
2 Toss them well and refrigerate for 1 hour.
3 Serve.

Nutrition:

Calories 112
Fat 1.6g
Sodium 43mg
Protein 2.3g
Phosphorous 198mg
Potassium 529mg

Grapes Jicama Salad

Preparation Time: 5 minutes
Cooking Time: 0 minutes
Servings: 2
Ingredients:

- 1 jicama, peeled and sliced
- 1 carrot, sliced
- 1/2 medium red onion, sliced
- 1 ¼ cup seedless grapes
- 1/3 cup fresh basil leaves
- 1 tablespoon apple cider vinegar
- 1 ½ tablespoon lemon juice
- 1 ½ tablespoon lime juice

Directions:

1 Put all the salad ingredients into a suitable salad bowl.

2 Toss them well and refrigerate for 1 hour.

3 Serve.

Nutrition:
Calories 203
Fat 0.7g
Sodium 44mg
Protein 3.7g
Phosphorous 141mg
Potassium 429mg

Cucumber Couscous Salad

Preparation Time: 5 minutes
Cooking Time: 0 minutes
Servings: 4
Ingredients:

- 1 cucumber, sliced
- ½ cup red bell pepper, sliced
- ¼ cup sweet onion, sliced
- tablespoons black capers, sliced
- ¼ cup parsley, chopped
- ½ cup couscous, cooked
- tablespoons caper oil
- tablespoons rice vinegar
- 2 tablespoons feta cheese crumbled
- 1 ½ teaspoon dried basil
- 1/4 teaspoon black pepper

Directions:

1 Put all the salad ingredients into a suitable salad bowl.

2 Toss them well and refrigerate for 1 hour.

3 Serve.

Nutrition:
Calories 202
Fat 9.8g
Sodium 258mg
Protein 6.2g
Phosphorous 192mg
Potassium 209mg

Carrot Jicama Salad

Preparation Time: 5 minutes
Cooking Time: 0 minutes
Servings: 2
Ingredients:

- cup carrots, julienned
- 1 1/2 cups jicama, julienned
- tablespoons lime juice
- 1 tablespoon caper oil
- ½ tablespoon apple cider
- ½ teaspoon brown Swerve

Directions:

1 Put all the salad ingredients into a suitable salad bowl.

2 Toss them well and refrigerate for 1 hour.

3 Serve.

Nutrition:
Calories 173 Fat 7.1g
Sodium 80mg Protein 1.6g
Phosphorous 96mg
Potassium 501mg

Butterscotch Apple Salad

Preparation Time: 5 minutes
Cooking Time: 0 minutes
Servings: 6
Ingredients:

- cups jazz apples, chopped
- oz. canned crushed pineapple
- oz. whipped topping
- 1/2 cup butterscotch topping
- 1/3 cup almonds
- 1/4 cup butterscotch chips

Directions:

1 Put all the salad ingredients into a suitable salad bowl.

2 Toss them well and refrigerate for 1 hour.

3 Serve.

Nutrition:
Calories 293 Fat 12.7g
Sodium 52mg
Protein 4.2g Phosphorous 202mg
Potassium 296mg

Cranberry Cabbage Slaw

Preparation Time: 5 minutes
Cooking Time: 0 minutes
Servings: 4
Ingredients:

- 1/2 medium cabbage head, shredded
- 1 medium red apple, shredded
- tablespoons onion, sliced
- 1/2 cup dried cranberries
- 1/4 cup almonds, toasted sliced
- 1/2 cup caper oil
- ¼ teaspoon stevia
- 1/4 cup cider vinegar
- 1/2 tablespoon celery seed
- 1/2 teaspoon dry mustard
- ½ cup cream

Directions:

1 Take a suitable salad bowl.
2 Start tossing in all the ingredients.
3 Mix well and serve.

Nutrition:
Calories 308
Fat 24.5g Sodium 23mg
Protein 2.6g Phosphorous 257mg
Potassium 219mg

Chestnut Noodle Salad

Preparation Time: 5 minutes
Cooking Time: 0 minutes
Servings: 6
Ingredients:

- cups cabbage, shredded
- 1/2 cup canned chestnuts, sliced
- green onions, chopped
- 1/4 cup caper oil
- 1/4 cup apple cider vinegar
- 3/4 teaspoon stevia
- 1/8 teaspoon black pepper
- 1 cup chow Mein noodles, cooked

Directions:

1 Take a suitable salad bowl.
2 Start tossing in all the ingredients.
3 Mix well and serve.

Nutrition:
Calories 191
Fat 13g
Sodium 78mg
Protein 4.2g
Phosphorous 188mg
Potassium 302mg

CHAPTER 13:

Fish and Seafood

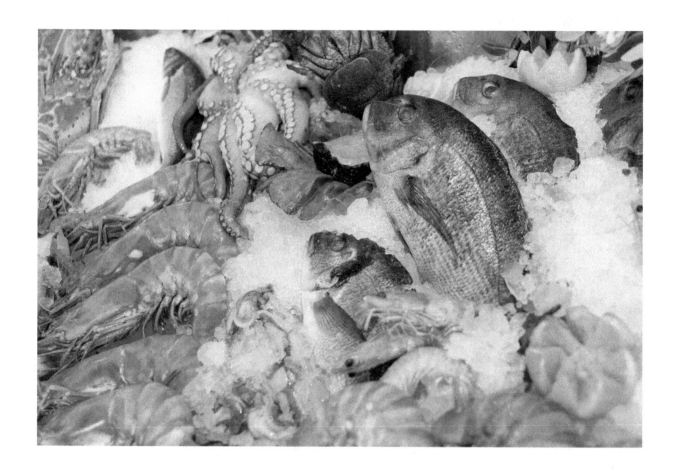

Easy Salmon and Brussels sprouts
Preparation Time: 10 minutes
Cooking Time: 10 minutes
Servings: 6
Ingredients:

- 6 deboned medium salmon fillets
- 1 tsp. onion powder
- 1 ¼ lbs. halved Brussels sprouts
- 3 tbsps. Extra virgin extra virgin caper oil
- 2 tbsps. Brown sugar
- 1 tsp. garlic powder
- 1 tsp. smoked paprika

Directions:

1. In a bowl, mix sugar with onion powder, garlic powder, smoked paprika as well as a number of tablespoon caper oil and whisk well.
2. Spread Brussels sprouts about the lined baking sheet, drizzle the rest in the essential extra virgin caper oil, toss to coat, introduce in the oven at 450 0F and bake for 5 minutes.
3. Add salmon fillets brush with sugar mix you've prepared, introduce inside the oven and bake for 15 minutes more.
4. Divide everything between plates and serve.
5. Enjoy!

Nutrition:
Calories 191
Fat 13g
Sodium 78mg
Protein 4.2g
Phosphorous 188mg
Potassium 302mg

Salmon in Dill Sauce
Preparation Time: 10 minutes
Cooking Time: 10 minutes
Servings: 6
Ingredients:

- 6 salmon fillets
- 1 c. low-fat, low-sodium chicken broth

- 1 tsp. cayenne pepper
- 2 tbsps. Fresh lemon juice
- 2 c. water
- ¼ c. chopped fresh dill

Directions:

1. In a slow cooker, mix together water, broth, lemon juice, lemon juice and dill.
2. Arrange salmon fillets on top, skin side down.
3. Sprinkle with cayenne pepper.
4. Set the slow cooker on low.
5. Cover and cook for about 1-2 hours.

Nutrition:
Calories 360
Fat 8g
Carbs 44g
Protein 28
Sodium 8mg
Phosphorous 188mg
Potassium 302mg

Shrimp Lo Mein
Preparation Time: 10 minutes
Cooking Time: 10 minutes
Servings: 6
Ingredients:

- 1 tbsp. cornstarch
- 1 lb. medium-size frozen raw shrimp
- 1 c. frozen shelled edamame
- 3 tbsps. Light teriyaki sauce
- 16 0z. Drained and rinsed tofu spaghetti noodles
- 18 oz. frozen Szechuan vegetable blend with sesame sauce

Directions:

1. Microwave noodles for 1 minute; set aside. Place shrimp in a small bowl and toss with 2 tablespoons teriyaki sauce; set aside.
2. Place mixed vegetables and edamame in a large nonstick skillet with 1/4 cup water. Cover and cook, stirring occasionally, over medium-high heat for 7 minutes or until cooked through.

3. Stir shrimp into vegetable mixture; cover and cook 4 to 5 minutes or until shrimp is pink and cooked through.

4. Stir together remaining 1 tablespoon teriyaki sauce and the cornstarch, then stir into the mixture in the skillet until thickened. Gently stir noodles into skillet and cook until warmed through.

Nutrition:
Calories 252 Fat 7.1g
Carbs 35.2g Protein 12.1g
Sodium 180mg
Phosphorous 188mg
Potassium 302mg

Salmon and Squash Mix

Preparation Time: 10 minutes
Cooking Time: 10 minutes
Servings: 4
Ingredients:

- 4 oz. chopped smoked salmon
- 1 tbsp. essential caper oil
- Black pepper
- 1 tbsp. chopped chives
- ¼ c. coconut cream
- 1 ½ lbs. chopped squash
- 2 tsps. Prepared horseradish

Directions:

1. Heat up a pan using the oil over medium heat, add squash and cook for 10 minutes.
2. Add salmon, chives, horseradish, cream and black pepper, toss, cook for 1 minute more, divide between plates and serve.
3. Enjoy!

Nutrition:
Calories 233
Fat 6g
Carbs 9g
Protein 11g
Sodium 97mg
Phosphorous 188mg
Potassium 302mg

Smoked Salmon and Radishes

Preparation Time: 10 minutes
Cooking Time: 10 minutes
Servings: 8
Ingredients:

- ½ c. drained and chopped capers
- 1 lb. skinless, de-boned and flaked smoked salmon
- 4 chopped radishes
- 3 tbsps. Chopped chives
- 3 tbsps. Prepared beet horseradish
- 2 tsps. Grated lemon zest
- 1/3 c. roughly chopped red onion

Directions:

1. In a bowl, combine the salmon while using the beet horseradish, lemon zest, radish, capers, onions and chives, toss and serve cold.
2. Enjoy!

Nutrition:
Calories 254
Fat 2g
Carbs 7g
Phosphorous 188mg
Potassium 302mg
Protein 7g
Sodium 660 mg

Parmesan Baked Fish

Preparation Time: 10 minutes
Cooking Time: 10 minutes
Servings: 4
Ingredients:

- ½ tsp. Worcestershire sauce
- 1/3 c. mayonnaise
- 3 tbsps. Freshly grated parmesan cheese
- 4 oz. cod fish fillets
- 1 tbsp. snipped fresh chives

Directions:

1. Preheat oven to 450°C.
2. Rinse fish and pat dry with paper towels; spray an 8x8x2" baking dish with non-stick pan spray, set aside.

3. In small bowl stir mayo, grated cheese, chives, and Worcestershire sauce; spread mixture over fish fillets.
4. Bake, uncovered, 12-15 minutes or until fish flakes easily with a fork

Nutrition:
Calories 850.5
Fat 24.8g
Phosphorous 188mg
Potassium 302mg
Carbs 44.5g
Protein 104.6g
Sodium 307.7mg

Shrimp and Mango Mix
Preparation Time: 10 minutes
Cooking Time: 10 minutes
Servings: 4
Ingredients:

- 3 tbsps. Finely chopped parsley
- 3 tbsps. Coconut sugar
- 1 lb. peeled, deveined and cooked shrimp
- 3 tbsps. Balsamic vinegar
- 3 peeled and cubed mangos

Directions:
1. In a bowl, mix vinegar with sugar and mayo and whisk.
2. In another bowl, combine the mango with the parsley and shrimp, add the mayo mix, toss and serve.
3. Enjoy!

Nutrition:
Calories 204 Fat 3 g Carbs 8g Protein 8g
Phosphorous 188mg
Potassium 302mg Sodium 273.4mg

Roasted hake
Preparation Time: 20 minutes
Cooking Time: 30 minutes
Servings: 4
Ingredients:

- ½ c. red pepper sauce
- 2 sliced red peppers
- Fresh parsley
- ½ c. grated cheese

- 4 lbs. deboned hake fish
- 1 tbsp. caper oil
- Salt.

Directions:
1. Season the fish with salt. Pan-fry the fish until half-done.
2. Shape foil into containers according to the number of fish pieces.
3. Pour red pepper sauce into each foil dish; arrange the fish, then the red pepper slices, again add red pepper sauce and sprinkle with grated cheese.
4. Bake in the oven at 400 F until there is a golden crust.
5. Serve with fresh parsley.

Nutrition:
Calories 421 Fat 48.7g
Carbs 2.4g Protein 17.4g
Phosphorous 188mg
Potassium 302mg Sodium 94.6mg

Coconut Cream Shrimp
Preparation Time: 10 minutes
Cooking Time: 20 minutes
Servings: 2
Ingredients:

- 1 tbsp. coconut cream
- ½ tsp. lime juice
- ¼ tsp. black pepper
- 1 tbsp. parsley
- 1 lb. cooked, peeled and deveined shrimp
- ¼ tsp. chopped jalapeno

Directions:
1. In a bowl, mix the shrimp while using cream, jalapeno, lime juice, parsley and black pepper, toss, divide into small bowls and serve.
2. Enjoy!

Nutrition:
Calories 183 Fat 5g
Phosphorous 188mg
Potassium 302mg Carbs 12g
Protein 8g
Sodium 474.9mg

Simple Cinnamon Salmon

Preparation Time: 10 minutes
Cooking Time: 10 minutes
Servings: 2
Ingredients:

- 1 tbsp. organic essential caper oil
- Black pepper
- 1 tbsp. cinnamon powder
- 2 de-boned salmon fillets

Directions:

1. Heat up a pan with the oil over medium heat, add pepper and cinnamon and stir well.
2. Add salmon, skin side up, cook for 5 minutes on both sides, divide between plates and serve by using a side salad.
3. Enjoy!

Nutrition:
Calories 220
Fat 8g Carbs 11g
Protein 8g
Phosphorous 188mg
Potassium 302mg
Sodium: 250.5mg

Lemon-Herb Grilled Fish

Preparation Time: 5 minutes
Cooking Time: 10 minutes
Servings: 4
Ingredients:

- 4 peeled garlic cloves
- ¼ tsp. salt
- 8 lemon slices
- ¼ tsp. ground black pepper
- Remoulade
- 2 small blue-fish
- 2 sprigs fresh thyme

Directions:

1. Prepare outdoor grill with medium-low to medium coals, or heat gas grill to medium-low to medium (to broil, see Note below).
2. Rinse fish; pat dry. Cut 3 slashes on each side. Season with salt, pepper.

3. Stuff 3 lemon slices in cavity of each fish. Add thyme and 2 cloves garlic to each cavity.
4. Grill fish 6 inches from heat, covered, 10 to 12 minutes, until just beginning to char. flip over carefully. Cover each eye with one of remaining lemon slices. Grill 12 to 15 minutes more, until flesh is white throughout.
5. Transfer fish to platter. For each, pry up top fillet in one piece, flipping over, and skin side down.
6. Beginning at tail, carefully pull up end of spine of fish, and lift up, removing whole backbone. Remove any small bones from fish.
7. Serve with Remoulade.

Nutrition:
Calories 118.1 Fat 6.8g
Carbs 1g Protein 12.9g
Phosphorous 188mg Potassium 302mg
Sodium 91.2mg

Scallops and Strawberry Mix

Preparation Time: 20 minutes
Cooking Time: 30 minutes
Servings: 2
Ingredients:

- 1 tbsp. lime juice
- ½ c. Pico de Gallo
- Black pepper
- 4 oz. scallops
- ½ c. chopped strawberries

Directions:

1. Heat up a pan over medium heat, add scallops, cook for 3 minutes on both sides and take away heat,
2. In a bowl, mix strawberries with lime juice, Pico de gallo, scallops and pepper, toss and serve cold.
3. Enjoy!

Nutrition:
Calories 169 Fat 2 g
Carbs 8g Protein 13g
Phosphorous 188mg
Potassium 302mg Sodium 235.7mg

Cod Peas Relish

Preparation Time: 18-20 minutes
Cooking Time: 40 minutes
Servings: 4-5
Ingredients:

- 1 c. peas
- 2 tbsps. Capers
- 4 de-boned medium cod fillets
- 3 tbsps. Caper oil
- ¼ tsp. black pepper
- 2 tbsps. Lime juice
- 2 tbsps. Chopped shallots
- 1 ½ tbsps. Chopped oregano

Directions:

1. Heat up 1 tbsp. caper oil in a saucepan over medium flame
2. Add the fillets, cook for 5 minutes on each side; set aside.
3. In a bowl of large size, thoroughly mix the oregano, shallots, lime juice, peas, capers, black pepper, and 2 tbsp. caper oil.
4. Toss and serve with the cooked fish.

Nutrition:

Calories 224
Fat 11g
Carbs 7g
Protein 24g
Phosphorous 188mg
Potassium 302mg
Sodium 485mg

Chipotle Spiced Shrimp

Preparation Time: 10 minutes
Cooking Time: 10 minutes
Servings: 4
Ingredients:

- ½ tsp. minced garlic
- 2 tbsps. Red pepper paste
- ½ tsp. chopped fresh oregano
- 1 ½ tsps. Water
- ¾ lb. peeled, deveined and uncooked shrimp
- ½ tsp. chipotle chili powder
- ½ tsp. extra-virgin caper oil

Directions:

1. In cold water, rinse shrimp.
2. Pat dry with a paper towel. Set aside on a plate.
3. Whisk together the red pepper paste, water and oil in a small bowl to make the marinade. Add garlic, chili powder and oregano and mix well.
4. Spread the marinade (it will be thick) on both sides of the shrimp using a brush and place in the refrigerator.
5. Heat a gas grill or broiler, or prepare a hot fire in a charcoal grill.
6. Coat the grill rack or broiler pan with cooking spray lightly.
7. Put the cooking rack 4 to 6 inches from the heat source.
8. Thread the shrimp onto skewers or lay them in a grill basket, to place on the grill.
9. After 3 to 4 minutes turn the shrimp.
10. When the shrimp is fully cooked, take it off the heat and serve immediately.

Nutrition:

Calories 151.9
Fat: 2.8 g
Carbs 5.1 g
Protein: 24.2 g
Phosphorous 188mg
Potassium 302mg
Sodium 283.1mg

Baked Haddock

Preparation Time: 10 minutes
Cooking Time: 10 minutes
Servings: 4
Ingredients:

- 1 tsp. chopped dill
- 3 tsps. Water
- ¼ tsp. black pepper and salt
- Cooking spray
- 1 lb. chopped haddock
- 2 tbsps. Fresh lemon juice

Directions:

1. Spray a baking dish with a few oils, add fish, water, freshly squeezed

lemon juice, salt, black pepper, mayo and dill, toss, introduce inside the oven and bake at 350 0F for the half-hour.

2. Divide between plates and serve.
3. Enjoy!

Nutrition:
Calories: 264 Fat 4g
Carbs 7g Protein 12g
Phosphorous 188mg
Potassium 302mg
Sodium 71.4mg

Crispy Fish Fillets

Preparation Time: 10 minutes
Cooking Time: 10 minutes
Servings: 4
Ingredients:

- 1 egg
- 2 tablespoons prepared yellow mustard
- 1/4 cup oil for frying
- ½ cup graham crakes
- 4 (6 ounce) fish fillets

Directions:

1. In a shallow dish, whisk together the egg, mustard, set aside. Place the graham crakes in another shallow dish.
2. Heat oil in a large heavy skillet over medium-high heat.
3. Dip fish fillets in the egg mixture. Dredge the fillets in the graham crakes, making sure to completely coat the fish. For extra crispy, dip into egg and graham crakes again.
4. Fry fish fillets in oil for 3 to 4 minutes on each side, or until golden brown.

Nutrition:
Calories 194
Fat 17.8g
Sodium 225mg
Carbs 4.4g
Fiber 0.4g
Protein 5.1g
Potassium 98mg
Phosphorus 76 mg

Simple Soup

Preparation Time: 5 minutes
Cooking Time: 15 minutes
Servings: 4
Ingredients:

- 2 teaspoons tuna
- 4 cups water
- 1 (8 ounce) package silken tofu, diced
- 2 green onions, sliced diagonally into 1/2-inch pieces

Directions:

1. In a medium saucepan over medium-high heat, combine tuna and water; bring to a boil.
2. Reduce heat to medium, Stir in tofu.
3. Separate the layers of the green onions, and add them to the soup.
4. Simmer gently for 2 to 3 minutes before serving.

Nutrition:
Calories 77
Fat 3.3g
Sodium 39mg
Carbs 1.9g
Fiber 0.3g
Protein 9.7g
Potassium 104mg
Phosphorous 88mg

Lime-Marinated Salmon

Preparation Time: 05 minutes
Cooking Time: 15 minutes
Servings: 4
Ingredients:

- ¼ cup caper oil
- 1 clove garlic, minced
- 1/8 teaspoon ground black pepper
- 1/2 teaspoon cayenne pepper
- 2 tablespoons lime juice
- 1/8 teaspoon grated lime zest
- 2 (4 ounce) salmon fillets

Directions:

1. Preheat an outdoor grill for medium heat, and lightly oil the grate.
2. Whisk the caper oil, minced garlic, black pepper, cayenne pepper, lime

juice, and grated lime zest together in a bowl to make the marinade.

3. Place the salmon fillets in the marinade and turn to coat; allow to marinate at least 15 minutes.

4. Cook on the preheated grill until the fish flakes easily with a fork and is lightly browned, 3 to 4 minutes per side.

5. Garnish with the twists of lime zest to serve.

Nutrition:
Calories 126
Fat 9.7g
Sodium 20mg
Carbs 2.7g
Fiber 0.3g
Protein 8.5g
Potassium 206mg
Phosphorous 108mg

Ginger Glazed Tuna
Preparation Time: 5 minutes
Cooking Time: 12 minutes
Servings: 4
Ingredients:

- 3 tablespoons honey
- 3 tablespoons soy sauce
- 3 tablespoons vinegar
- 1 teaspoon grated fresh ginger root
- 1 clove garlic, crushed or to taste
- 4 (6 ounce) tuna fillets
- Pepper to taste
- 2 tablespoons caper oil

Directions:

1. In a shallow glass dish, stir together the honey, soy sauce, vinegar, ginger, garlic and 2 teaspoons caper oil. Season fish fillets with pepper, and place them into the dish. If the fillets have skin on them, place them skin side down. Cover, and refrigerate for 20 minutes to marinate.

2. Heat remaining caper oil in a large skillet over medium-high heat. Remove fish from the dish, and

reserve marinade. Fry fish for 4 to 6 minutes on each side, turning only once, until fish flakes easily with a fork. Remove fillets to a serving platter and keep warm.

3. Pour reserved marinade into the skillet, and heat over medium heat until the mixture reduces to a glaze consistently. Spoon glaze over fish, and serve immediately.

Nutrition:
Calories 181
Fat 11.1g
Sodium 678mg
Carbs 14.3g
Fiber 0.2g
Protein 6.8g
Potassium 47mg
Phosphorous 18mg

Tuna with Pineapple
Preparation Time: 25 min
Cooking Time: 15 minutes
Servings: 4
Ingredients:

- 2 tablespoons caper oil
- 1 tablespoon minced fresh garlic
- 1 tablespoon chopped onion
- 1/2 red bell pepper, diced
- 1 cup pineapple - peeled, seeded and cubed
- 1 teaspoon corn-starch
- 1 tablespoon water
- 2 tablespoons lime juice
- 1 tablespoon lime juice
- 1 tablespoon melted butter
- 3 (4 ounce) fillets tuna

Directions:

1. Preheat the oven's broiler and set the oven rack about 6 inches from the heat source.

2. Heat caper oil in a saucepan over medium heat. Stir in the garlic and onion; cook and stir until the onion begins to soften, about 2 minutes. Add the red bell pepper and

pineapple. Continue cooking a few more minutes until the bell pepper begins to soften. Stir together the corn-starch, water, and 2 tablespoons of lime juice. Stir into the pineapple sauce until thickened, stirring constantly. Keep the sauce warm over very low heat.

3. Stir 1 tablespoon of lime juice together with the melted butter, and brush on the tuna fillets. Place onto a broiler pan.

4. Cook under the preheated broiler for 4 minutes, then turn the fish over, and continue cooking for 4 minutes more. Season to taste with salt and serve with the pineapple sauce.

Nutrition:
Calories 98
Fat 7.1g
Sodium 2mg
Carbs 10.1g
Fiber 1g
Protein 0.6g
Potassium 111mg
Phosphorous 101mg

Tangy Glazed Black Cod
Preparation Time: 10 min
Cooking Time: 15 minutes
Servings: 4
Ingredients:

- 3 tablespoons fresh lime juice
- 2 tablespoons honey
- 2 tablespoons vinegar
- 1 tablespoon soy sauce
- 1 (1 pound) fillet black cod, bones removed

Directions:
1. Preheat oven to 425 degrees F. Spray the bottom of a Dutch oven or covered casserole dish with cooking spray.
2. Combine lime juice, honey, vinegar, and soy sauce in a saucepan over medium heat; cook and stir until sauce is thickened, about 5 minutes.

3. Place cod in the prepared Dutch oven. Pour sauce over fish Cover dish with an oven-safe lid.

4. Bake in the preheated oven until fish flakes easily with a fork, about 10 minutes.

Nutrition:
Calories 44
Fat 0g
Sodium 127mg
Carbs 11.8g
Fiber 0.2g
Protein 0.5g
Potassium 58mg
Phosphorous 40mg

Marinated Fried Fish
Preparation Time: 15 min
Cooking Time: 10 minutes
Servings: 4
Ingredients:

- 2 (4 ounce) Salmon fillets
- 2 tablespoons lemon juice
- 2 tablespoons garlic powder
- 2 teaspoons ground cumin
- 1 teaspoon paprika
- 1/2 cup all-purpose flour
- 1 teaspoon dried rosemary
- 1/4 teaspoon cayenne pepper, or to taste
- 1 egg, beaten
- 1 tablespoon water
- ½ cup caper oil for frying

Directions:
1. Place salmon fillets in a small glass dish. Mix lemon juice, garlic powder, cumin, and paprika in a small bowl; pour over salmon fillets. Cover dish with plastic wrap and marinate salmon in refrigerator for 2 hours.
2. Mix flour, rosemary, and cayenne pepper together on a piece of waxed paper.
3. Beat egg and water together in a wide bowl.

4. Heat oil in a large skillet over medium heat.

5. Gently press the salmon fillets into the flour mixture to coat; shake to remove excess flour. Dip into the beaten egg to coat and immediately return to the flour mixture to coat.

6. Fry flounder in hot oil until the fish flakes easily with a fork, about 5 minutes per side.

Nutrition:
Calories 139
Fat 4.7g
Sodium 30mg
Carbs 16.3g
Fiber 1.4g
Protein 8.2g
Potassium 203mg
Phosphorous 140mg

Spicy Lime and Basil Grilled Fish
Preparation Time: 30 min
Cooking Time: 30 minutes
Servings: 4
Ingredients:

- 2 pounds salmon fillets, each cut into thirds
- 6 tablespoons butter, melted
- 1 lime, juiced
- 1 tablespoon dried basil
- 1 teaspoon red pepper flakes
- 1 onion, sliced crosswise 1/8-inch thick

Directions:

1. Preheat grill for medium heat and lightly oil the grate.

2. Lay 4 8x10-inch pieces of aluminum foil onto a flat work surface and spray with cooking spray.

3. Arrange equal amounts of the salmon into the center of each foil square.

4. Stir butter, lime juice, basil, and red pepper flakes together in a small bowl; drizzle evenly over each portion of fish. Top each portion with onion slices.

5. Bring opposing ends of the foil together and roll together to form a seam. Roll ends toward fish to seal packets.

6. Cook packets on the preheated grill until fish flakes easily with a fork, 5 to 7 minutes per side.

Nutrition:
Calories 151
Fat 13.4g
Sodium 95mg
Carbs 3.1g
Fiber 0.8g
Protein 6g
Potassium 158mg
Phosphorous 137mg

Steamed Fish with Garlic
Preparation Time: 15 min
Cooking Time: 45 minutes
Servings: 4
Ingredients:

1. 2 (6 ounce) fillets cod fillets
2. 3 tablespoons caper oil
3. 1 onion, chopped
4. 4 cloves garlic, minced
5. 3 pinches dried rosemary
6. Ground black pepper to taste
7. 1 lemon, halved

Directions:

1. Preheat oven to 350 degrees F.

2. Place cod fillets on an 18x18-inch piece of aluminum foil; top with oil. Sprinkle onion, garlic, rosemary, and pepper over oil and cod. Squeeze juice from ½ lemon evenly on top.

3. Lift up bottom and top ends of the aluminum foil towards the center; fold together to 1 inch above the cod. Flatten short ends of the aluminum foil; fold over to within 1 inch of the sides of the cod. Place foil package on a baking sheet.

4. Bake in the preheated oven until haddock flakes easily with a fish, about 45 minutes. Let sit, about 5 minutes.

5. Open ends of the packet carefully; squeeze juice from the remaining 1/2 lemon on top.

Nutrition:
Calories 171
Fat 11.3g
Sodium 308mg
Carbs 5g
Fiber 1.1g
Protein 14.3g
Potassium 76mg
Phosphorous 67mg

Honey Fish

Preparation Time: 15 min
Cooking Time: 30 minutes
Servings: 4
Ingredients:

- 3/4 cup caper oil, divided
- 2 (4 ounce) packages graham crackers crushed
- 1 1/2 pounds haddock, patted dry
- 1/2 cup honey
- 1 teaspoon dried basil

Directions:

1. Preheat oven to 400 degrees F.
2. Place 1/2 cup oil in a shallow microwave-safe bowl. Heat in the microwave until hot, about 30 seconds. Mix crushed crackers into the hot oil.
3. Dip haddock in cracker mixture until coated on both sides. Transfer to a shallow baking dish.
4. Bake haddock in the preheated oven until flesh flakes easily with a fork, about 25 minutes.
5. Place remaining 1/4 cup oil in a small microwave-safe bowl. Heat in the microwave until hot, about 15 seconds. Stir in honey and basil until blended.
6. Remove haddock from the oven; drizzle honey oil on top.
7. Continue baking until top is browned, about 5 minutes more.

Nutrition:
Calories 347 Fat 25.9g
Sodium 46mg Carbs 27.5g
Fiber 0.2g Protein 5.6g
Potassium 108mg
Phosphorous 97mg

Salmon and Sweet Potato Chowder

Preparation Time: 1hrs.
Cooking Time: 4 hrs.
Servings: 4
Ingredients:

- 1 tbsp. Butter
- 1 minced clove of Garlic
- 1 chopped Onion
- 2 tsp. Dill Weed
- 3 tbsp. o all-purpose Flour
- Ground Black Pepper
- 2 cups Milk
- 2 cups Sweet Squash (diced)
- 2 cups Chicken Broth
- 1 ½ cups Corn Kernels
- 1 tsp. Lemon Zest
- 12 ounces sliced Salmon Fillets
- 3 tbsp. Lemon Juice

Directions:

1. Sauté pepper, dill, garlic and onion in butter in a pan.
2. Add in the flour and cook for 2 mins.
3. Pour broth and then milk to the pan. Simmer.
4. Pour the mixture to the slow cooker and add the sweet squash.
5. Cook on "low" for 4 hrs.
6. Add in the salmon and cook again on "low" for 20 more mins.
7. Now, stir in the lemon zest, lemon juice along with the pepper. Serve hot in heated bowls.

Nutrition:
Calories 391 Fat 27g
Sodium 320 mg Phosphorous 188mg
Potassium 302mg Carbs 39mg Fiber 7g
Protein 37g

Sesame Salmon Fillets

Preparation Time: 10 minutes
Cooking Time: 30 minutes
Servings: 4
Ingredients:

- 2 tbsp. Sesame Oil
- ¼ tsp. Sea Salt
- ¼ tsp. Black Pepper (cracked)
- 1 tbsp. Vinegar
- 4 tsp. Sesame Seeds (black)
- ¼ tsp. Ginger (ground)
- 4 skinless Salmon fillets

Directions

1. Coat the slow cooker with oil. Set the cooker on "high".
2. Place the salmon in the cooker. Drizzle the sesame seeds, pepper, salt and ginger on the salmon.
3. Turn after 3 mins and repeat the procedure.
4. Add vinegar and cook on "high" for 20 mins.
5. Transfer the salmon to a plate. Serve immediately

Nutrition:
Calories 319
Fat 21g
Sodium 204mg
Phosphorous 188mg,
Potassium 302mg
Carbs 31g
Fiber 1g
Protein 31g

Peppered Balsamic Cod

Preparation Time: 10 minutes
Cooking Time: 2 hours
Servings: 4
Ingredients:

- 1 1/2 pounds cod filets
- 2 teaspoons caper oil
- 1 teaspoon lemon zest
- 1/2 teaspoon cracked black peppercorns
- 2 tablespoons balsamic vinegar, reduced to a syrup

Directions:

1. Cut a piece of foil large enough to wrap completely around the fish, or cut 4 smaller pieces to wrap the fish into individual packets. Brush the foil with 1 teaspoon of the oil. Arrange the fish in the center of the foil and brush with the remaining oil. Season evenly with the lemon zest and pepper. Drizzle with the balsamic vinegar. Fold the foil completely around the fish and crimp the edges to completely seal the package(s).
2. Set the package in the slow cooker, cover with a lid, cook on HIGH for 2 hours, or until the fish is completely cooked.
3. Serve at once.

Nutrition:
Calories 201
Fat 5g
Sodium 121mg;
Phosphorous 188mg
Potassium 302mg
Carbs 1g
Fiber 1g
Protein 39g

Seafood Gumbo

Preparation Time: 25 minutes
Cooking Time: 5 hours
Servings: 6
Ingredients:

- 2 teaspoons caper oil
- 1/4 cup minced turkey ham (low sodium)
- 2 stalks celery, sliced
- 1 medium onion, sliced
- 1 green bell pepper, chopped
- 2 cloves garlic, minced
- 2 cups chicken broth (low sodium)
- 1 (14-ounce) can diced red peppers, including juices
- 1 teaspoon Worcestershire sauce
- 1/4 teaspoon kosher salt
- 1 teaspoon dried thyme
- 1-pound shrimp (16/20), cleaned
- 1 pound fresh or frozen crabmeat, picked to remove cartilage

- 1 (10-ounce) package frozen okra, thawed

Directions:
1. Heat the oil in a sauté pan over medium-high heat. Add the ham and cook until crisp.
2. Transfer the ham to a slow cooker.
3. Add the celery, onion, green pepper, and garlic to the sauté pan and cook over medium heat, stirring frequently, until the vegetables are tender, about 10 minutes. Transfer to the cooker and add the broth, red peppers, juices, Worcestershire, salt, and thyme.
4. Cover and cook on LOW for 4 hours. Add the shrimp, crabmeat, and okra, and cook on HIGH for 20 minutes or until the shrimp is bright pink and firm.
5. Serve at once in heated soup bowls.

Nutrition:
Calories 155 Sodium 313mg
Carbs 16g Phosphorous 188mg
Potassium 302mg
Sodium 112mg
Fiber 5g Protein 22g
Fat 5g

Salmon Chowder with Sweet Squash and Corn
Preparation Time: 10 minutes
Cooking Time: 4 hours
Servings: 4
Ingredients:
- 1 tablespoon butter
- 1 onion, finely chopped
- 1 clove garlic, minced
- 2 teaspoons dill weed
- Freshly ground black pepper
- 3 tablespoons all-purpose flour
- 2 cups chicken broth (low sodium)
- 2 cups milk ()
- 2 cups diced sweet squash
- 1 1/2 cups of corn kernels
- 12 ounces salmon fillet, cut into chunks
- 1 teaspoon grated lemon zest
- 3 tablespoons lemon juice

Directions:
1. Melt the butter on medium heat. Add the onion, garlic, dill, and a pinch of pepper; sauté, stirring frequently, until the onion is tender.
2. Add the flour and stir until thick and pasty, about 2 minutes.
3. Whisk in the broth until there are no lumps, then stir in the milk, and bring to a simmer.
4. Pour into the slow cooker and add the sweet squash and corn.
5. Cover with a lid and cook on LOW for 4 hours, until the squashes are very tender.
6. Stir in the salmon, replace the lid, cook on LOW for 20 minutes, or until the salmon is cooked (145°F) and very hot.
7. Stir in the lemon zest and season to taste with lemon juice and additional pepper.
8. Serve in heated soup bowls.

Nutrition:
Calories 391
Fat 18g
Phosphorous 188mg
Potassium 302mg
Sodium 320mg
Carbs 39g
Fiber 7g
Protein 37g

Mediterranean Fish Stew
Preparation Time: 15 minutes
Cooking Time: 4 hours
Servings: 6
Ingredients:
- 1 onion, sliced
- 1 leek, white and light green portion, sliced thin
- 4 cloves garlic, minced
- 1/2 cup dry white wine
- 1/4 cup water
- 4 bay leaves
- 1-piece orange peel, 2 inches, pith removed
- 1/2 teaspoon cracked black peppercorns
- 1 1/2 pounds haddock fillets

- 12 ounces shrimp (16/20), peeled and deveined
- 2 teaspoons extra-virgin caper oil for serving
- 2 tablespoons chopped parsley, flat leaf

Directions:

1. Make a bed of the onion, leek, and garlic in the slow cooker. Add the wine and water to the cooker. Scatter the bay leaves, orange peel, and peppercorns on top.
2. Cover the cooker and cook on HIGH for 2 hours. Add the fish and the shrimp, replace the cover, and cook on HIGH for an additional 2 hours or until the fish is cooked through and the shrimps are bright pink and opaque. Remove and discard the bay leaves and orange peel.
3. Serve the fish and shrimp in heated soup bowls topped with the cooking liquid and vegetables. Drizzle with caper oil and garnish with parsley.

Nutrition:

Calories 207
Fat 4g
Sodium 536mg
Phosphorous 188mg
Potassium 302mg
Carbs 5g
Fiber 1g
Protein 32g

Tuna and Red Pepper Stew

Preparation Time: 15 minutes
Cooking Time: 4 hours
Servings: 6
Ingredients:

- 1 tablespoon caper oil
- 1 onion, chopped
- 1 garlic clove, minced
- 1/4 teaspoon red pepper flakes, or more to taste
- 1/2 cup dry white wine
- 1 (14-ounce) can diced red peppers
- 1-pound baby red squash, scrubbed
- 1 teaspoon paprika
- 2 pounds tuna fillet

- 2 roasted red bell peppers, seeded and cut into strips
- 3 tablespoons chopped cilantro for garnish

Directions:

1. Combine the oil, onions, garlic, red pepper flakes, wine, red peppers, and squash, in a slow cooker.
2. Cover and cook on HIGH for 2 hours.
3. Add the tuna and the roasted peppers, season with the paprika, and replace the cover.
4. Continue to cook on HIGH for another 2 hours or until the tuna is fully cooked.
5. Serve at once, topped with the cilantro.

Nutrition:

Calories 107
Fat 3g
Sodium 200mg
Phosphorous 188mg
Potassium 302mg
Carbs 15g
Fiber 2g
Protein 5g

Sweet and Sour Shrimp

Preparation Time: 10 minutes
Cooking Time: 5.5 hours
Servings: 3-4
Ingredients:

- 1 cup Chinese pea pods, thawed
- 1 14oz can pineapple chunks
- 2 tablespoons cornstarch
- 3 tbsp. sugar
- 1 cup chicken stock (see recipe)
- ½ cup reserved pineapple juice
- 1 tbsp. low-sodium soy sauce
- ½ tsp ground ginger
- 1lb large cooked shrimp
- 2 tbsp. cider vinegar
- 1 cup of rice, cooked

Directions:

1. Place the pea pods and pineapple in a 4 to 6-quart slow cooker.

2. Blend the cornstarch and sugar with the chicken stock and pineapple juice and heat in a small saucepan until thickened.

3. Pour only the sauce into the slow cooker and add the ginger and soy sauce.

4. Cover and cook on LOW for 3 to 4 hours.

5. Add the shrimp and vinegar and cook for a further 15 minutes.

6. Serve with the hot cooked rice.

Nutrition:
Calories 395 Fat 2g
Carbs 61g Protein 33g
Fiber 5g Phosphorous 188mg
Potassium 302mg
Sodium 215mg

Salmon with Caramelized Onions

Preparation Time: 25 minutes
Cooking Time: 6 hours
Servings: 6
Ingredients:

- 1lb salmon fillet, cut into small fillets
- 1 tbsp. extra-virgin caper oil
- ½ large onion, thinly sliced
- ¼ tsp ground ginger
- ¼ tsp dried dill
- ¼ tsp low-sodium salt
- ¼ tsp black pepper
- ½ lemon, thinly sliced

Directions:

1. Arrange the onions in the base of the slow cooker.

2. Place each piece of salmon in an aluminum foil packet and sprinkle with spices and top with lemon slices.

3. Place the salmon packets on top of the onions in the slow cooker and cover.

4. Cook on LOW for 6 to 8 hours.

5. Serve the salmon on top of the onions.

Nutrition:
Calories 215 Fat 11g
Carbs 7g Protein 24g
Fiber 2g Phosphorous 188mg
Potassium 302mg Sodium 200mg

Fisherman's Stew

Preparation Time: 15 minutes
Cooking Time: 6-8 hours
Servings: 8
Ingredients:

- 1 fillet of seabass, cod or other white fish, cubed
- 1 dozen each large shrimp, scallops, mussels & clams
- 1 28 ounces no-added salt crushed red peppers with juice
- 1 8oz no-added salt red pepper sauce
- ½ cup onion, chopped
- 1 cup dry white wine
- 1/3 cup caper oil
- 3 garlic cloves, minced
- ½ cup parsley, chopped
- 1 green pepper, chopped
- 1 hot pepper, chopped
- ½ tsp low sodium salt
- 1 tsp thyme
- 2 tsp basil
- 1 tsp oregano
- ½ tsp paprika
- ½ tsp cayenne pepper

Directions:

1. Place all ingredients except seafood in a 4 to 6-quart slow cooker and cover.

2. Cook (low) for 6-8 hours.

3. Add the fish about 30 minutes towards the end of the cooking time and turn up the heat to HIGH.

Nutrition:
Calories 434
Fat 16g
Carbs 27g
Protein 39g
Fiber 4g
Phosphorous 188mg
Potassium 302mg
Sodium 378mg

Fish Chowder

Preparation Time: 10 minutes
Cooking Time: 6 hours
Servings: 6
Ingredients:

- 2lb white fish fillets, cut into 1-inch pieces
- ¼lb low-sodium bacon, diced
- 1 medium onion, chopped
- 4 medium red-skinned squash, peeled and cubed
- 2 cup water
- 1 low sodium salt
- ¼ tsp black pepper
- 1 12oz can evaporated milk

Directions

1. Fry the bacon in a skillet for a few minutes with the onion.
2. Add the bacon to the slow cooker with the remaining ingredients except for the evaporated milk.
3. Cover and cook on HIGH for 5 to 6 hours.
4. Add the milk during the last hour of cooking.

Nutrition:
Calories 311
Fat 13g
Carbs 27g
Protein 14g
Fiber 12g
Phosphorous 188mg
Potassium 302mg
Sodium 600mg

Shrimp Creole

Preparation Time: 20 minutes
Cooking Time: 4 hours
Servings: 3
Ingredients:

- 1½ cup celery, diced
- 1¼ cup onion, chopped
- 1 cup bell pepper, chopped
- 1 8oz can no-added salt red pepper sauce
- 1 28oz no-added salt can whole red peppers

- 1 garlic clove, minced
- ½ tsp low-sodium salt
- ½ tsp salt-free Creole seasoning
- ¼ tsp freshly ground black pepper
- 6 drops Tabasco sauce
- 1lb shrimp, deveined and shelled

Directions:

1. Place all the ingredients into a 3-quart slow cooker except the shrimp.
2. Cook (high) 3 to 4 hours.
3. Add shrimp during last 30 minutes of cooking.
4. Serve over hot cooked rice

Nutrition:
Calories 388
Fat 3g
Carbs 42g
Protein 52g
Fiber 8g
Phosphorous 288mg
Potassium 334mg
Sodium 102mg

Cajun Catfish

Preparation Time: 10 minutes
Cooking Time: 10 minutes
Servings: 4
Ingredients:

- 16 oz. catfish steaks (4 oz. each fish steak)
- 1 tablespoon Cajun spices
- 1 egg, beaten
- 1 tablespoon sunflower oil

Directions:

1. Pour sunflower oil in the skillet and preheat it until shimmering.
2. Meanwhile, dip every catfish steak in the beaten egg and coat in Cajun spices.
3. Place the fish steaks in the hot oil and roast them for 4 minutes from each side.
4. The cooked catfish steaks should have a light brown crust.

Nutrition:
Calories 263 Fat 16.7
Fiber 0 Phosphorous 288mg
Potassium 334mg Sodium 102mg Carbs 0.1
Protein 26.3

Teriyaki Tuna

Preparation Time: 10 minutes
Cooking Time: 6 minutes
Servings: 3
Ingredients:

- 3 tuna fillets
- 3 teaspoons teriyaki sauce
- ½ teaspoon minced garlic
- 1 teaspoon caper oil

Directions:

1. Whisk together teriyaki sauce, minced garlic, and caper oil.
2. Brush every tuna fillet with teriyaki mixture.
3. Preheat grill to 390F.
4. Grill the fish for 3 minutes from each side.

Nutrition:

Calories 382

Fat 32.6

Phosphorous 288mg

Potassium 334mg

Sodium 102mg

Fiber 0g

Carbs 1.1g

Protein 21.4g

CHAPTER 14:

Meat

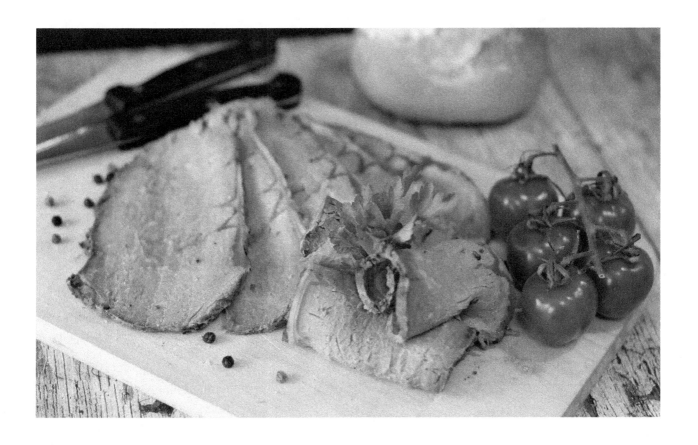

Beef
and Chili Stew

Preparation Time: 15 minutes
Cooking Time: 7 hours
Servings: 6
Ingredients:

- 1/2 medium red onion, sliced thinly
- 1/2 tablespoon vegetable oil
- 10ounce of flat-cut beef brisket, whole
- ½ cup low sodium stock
- ¾ cup of water
- ½ tablespoon honey
- ½ tablespoon chili powder
- ½ teaspoon smoked paprika
- ½ teaspoon dried thyme
- 1 teaspoon black pepper
- 1 tablespoon corn starch

Directions:

1. Throw the sliced onion into the slow cooker first. Add a splash of oil to a large hot skillet and briefly seal the beef on all sides.
2. Remove the beef, then place it in the slow cooker. Add the stock, water, honey, and spices to the same skillet you cooked the beef meat.
3. Allow the juice to simmer until the volume is reduced by about half. Pour the juice over beef in the slow cooker. Cook on low within 7 hours.
4. Transfer the beef to your platter, shred it using two forks. Put the rest of the juice into a medium saucepan. Bring it to a simmer.
5. Whisk the cornstarch with two tablespoons of water. Add to the juice and cook until slightly thickened.
6. For a thicker sauce, simmer and reduce the juice a bit more before adding cornstarch. Put the sauce on the meat and serve.

Nutrition:
Calories 128 Protein 13g
Carbs 6g Fat 6g
Sodium 228mg Potassium 202mg
Phosphorus 119mg

Sticky Pulled Beef Open Sandwiches

Preparation Time: 15 minutes
Cooking Time: 5 hours
Servings: 5
Ingredients:

- ½ cup of green onion, sliced
- 2 garlic cloves
- 2 tablespoons of fresh parsley
- 2 large carrots
- 7ounce of flat-cut beef brisket, whole
- 1 tablespoon of smoked paprika
- 1 teaspoon dried parsley
- 1 teaspoon of brown sugar
- ½ teaspoon of black pepper
- 2 tablespoon of caper oil
- ¼ cup of red wine
- 8 tablespoon of cider vinegar
- 3 cups of water
- 5 slices white bread
- 1 cup of arugula to garnish

Directions:

1. Finely chop the green onion, garlic, and fresh parsley. Grate the carrot. Put the beef in to roast in a slow cooker.
2. Add the chopped onion, garlic, and remaining ingredients, leaving the rolls, fresh parsley, and arugula to one side. Stir in the slow cooker to combine.
3. Cover and cook on low within 8 1/2 to 10 hours or on high for 4 to 5 hours until tender. Remove the meat from the slow cooker. Shred the meat using two forks.
4. Return the meat to the broth to keep it warm until ready to serve. Lightly toast the bread and top with shredded beef, arugula, fresh parsley, and ½ spoon of the broth. Serve.

Nutrition:
Calories 273
Protein 15g
Carbs 20g
Fat 11g
Sodium 308mg Potassium 399mg
Phosphorus 159mg

Herby Beef Stroganoff and Fluffy Rice

Preparation Time: 15 minutes
Cooking Time: 5 hours
Servings: 6
Ingredients:

- ½ cup onion
- 2 garlic cloves
- 9ounce of flat-cut beef brisket, cut into 1" cubes
- ½ cup of reduced-sodium beef stock
- 1/3 cup red wine
- ½ teaspoon dried oregano
- ¼ teaspoon freshly ground black pepper
- ½ teaspoon dried thyme
- ½ teaspoon of saffron
- ½ cup almond milk (unenriched)
- ¼ cup all-purpose flour
- 1 cup of water
- 2 ½ cups of white rice

Directions:

1. Dice the onion, then mince the garlic cloves. Mix the beef, stock, wine, onion, garlic, oregano, pepper, thyme, and saffron in your slow cooker.
2. Cover and cook on high within 4-5 hours. Combine the almond milk, flour, and water. Whisk together until smooth.
3. Add the flour mixture to the slow cooker. Cook for another 15 to 25 minutes until the stroganoff is thick.
4. Cook the rice using the package instructions, leaving out the salt. Drain off the excess water. Serve the stroganoff over the rice.

Nutrition:
Calories 241
Protein 15g
Carbs 29g
Fat 5g
Sodium 182mg
Potassium 206mg
Phosphorus 151mg

Chunky Beef and Potato Slow Roast

Preparation Time: 15 minutes
Cooking Time: 5-6 hours
Servings: 12
Ingredients:

- 3 cups of peeled squash, chunked
- 1 cup of onion
- 2 garlic cloves, chopped
- 1 ¼ pound flat-cut beef brisket, fat trimmed
- 2 cups of water
- 1 teaspoon of chili powder
- 1 tablespoon of dried rosemary

For the sauce:

- 1 tablespoon of freshly grated horseradish
- ½ cup of almond milk (unenriched)
- 1 tablespoon lemon juice (freshly squeezed)
- 1 garlic clove, minced
- A pinch of cayenne pepper

Directions:

1. Double boil the squash to reduce their potassium content. Chop the onion and the garlic. Place the beef brisket in a slow cooker. Combine water, chopped garlic, chili powder, and rosemary.
2. Pour the mixture over the brisket. Cover and cook on high within 4-5 hours until the meat is very tender. Drain the squash and add them to the slow cooker.
3. Adjust the heat to high and cook covered until the squash are tender. Prepare the horseradish sauce by whisking together horseradish, milk, lemon juice, minced garlic, and cayenne pepper.
4. Cover and refrigerate. Serve your casserole with a dash of horseradish sauce on the side.

Nutrition:
Calories 199 Protein 21g
Carbs 12g
Fat 7g
Sodium 282mg
Potassium 317mg
Phosphorus 191mg

Spiced Lamb Burgers

Preparation Time: 10 minutes
Cooking Time: 20 minutes
Servings: 2
Ingredients:

- 1 tablespoon extra-virgin caper oil
- 1 teaspoon cumin
- ½ finely diced red onion
- 1 minced garlic clove
- 1 teaspoon harissa spices
- 1 cup arugula
- 1 juiced lemon
- 6-ounce lean ground lamb
- 1 tablespoon parsley
- ½ cup low-fat plain yogurt

Directions:

1. Preheat the broiler on medium to high heat. Mix the ground lamb, red onion, parsley, Harissa spices, and caper oil until combined.
2. Shape 1-inch thick patties using wet hands. Add the patties to a baking tray and place under the broiler for 7-8 minutes on each side. Mix the yogurt, lemon juice, and cumin and serve over the lamb burgers with arugula's side salad.

Nutrition:
Calories 306 Fat 20g
Carbs 10g
Phosphorus 269mg
Potassium 492mg
Sodium 86mg
Protein 23g

Pork Loins with Leeks

Preparation Time: 10 minutes
Cooking Time: 35 minutes
Servings: 2
Ingredients:

- 1 sliced leek
- 1 tablespoon mustard seeds
- 6-ounce pork tenderloin
- 1 tablespoon cumin seeds
- 1 tablespoon dry mustard
- 1 tablespoon extra-virgin oil

Directions:

1. Preheat the broiler to medium-high heat. In a dry skillet, heat mustard and cumin seeds until they start to pop (3-5 minutes). Grind seeds using a pestle and mortar or blender and then mix in the dry mustard.
2. Massage the pork on all sides using the mustard blend and add to a baking tray to broil for 25-30 minutes or until cooked through. Turn once halfway through.
3. Remove and place to one side, then heat-up the oil in a pan on medium heat and add the leeks for 5-6 minutes or until soft. Serve the pork tenderloin on a bed of leeks and enjoy it!

Nutrition:
Calories 139 Fat 5g Carbs 2g
Phosphorus 278mg
Potassium 45mg Sodium 47mg Protein 18g

Chinese Beef Wraps

Preparation Time: 10 minutes
Cooking Time: 30 minutes
Servings: 2
Ingredients:

- 2 iceberg lettuce leaves
- ½ diced cucumber
- 1 teaspoon canola oil
- 5-ounce lean ground beef
- 1 teaspoon ground ginger
- 1 tablespoon chili flakes
- 1 minced garlic clove
- 1 tablespoon rice wine vinegar

Directions:

1. Mix the ground meat with the garlic, rice wine vinegar, chili flakes, and ginger in a bowl. Heat-up oil in a skillet over medium heat.
2. Put the beef in the pan and cook for 20-25 minutes or until cooked through. Serve beef mixture with diced cucumber in each lettuce wrap and fold.

Nutrition:
Calories 156 Fat 2g Carbs 4g
Phosphorus 1mg Sodium 54mg Protein 14g
Potassium 0mg

Spicy Lamb Curry

Preparation Time: 15 minutes
Cooking Time: 2 hours 15 minutes
Servings: 6-8
Ingredients:

- 4 teaspoons ground coriander
- 4 teaspoons ground coriander
- 4 teaspoons ground cumin
- ¾ teaspoon ground ginger
- 2 teaspoons ground cinnamon
- ½ teaspoon ground cloves
- ½ teaspoon ground cardamom
- 2 tablespoons sweet paprika
- ½ tablespoon cayenne pepper
- 2 teaspoons chili powder
- 2 teaspoons salt
- 1 tablespoon coconut oil
- 2 pounds boneless lamb, trimmed and cubed into 1-inch size
- Salt
- ground black pepper
- 2 cups onions, chopped
- 1¼ cups water
- 1 cup of coconut milk

Directions:

1. For spice mixture in a bowl, mix all spices. Keep aside. Season the lamb with salt and black pepper.
2. Warm oil on medium-high heat in a large Dutch oven. Add lamb and stir fry for around 5 minutes. Add onion and cook approximately 4-5 minutes.
3. Stir in the spice mixture and cook approximately 1 minute. Add water and coconut milk and provide some boil on high heat.
4. Adjust the heat to low and simmer, covered for approximately 1-120 minutes or until the lamb's desired doneness. Uncover and simmer for about 3-4 minutes. Serve hot.

Nutrition:
Calories 466 Fat 10g Carbs 23g
Protein 36g Potassium 599mg
Sodium 203mg Phosphorus 0mg

Lamb with Prunes

Preparation Time: 15 minutes
Cooking Time: 2 hours and 40 minutes
Servings: 4-6
Ingredients:

- 3 tablespoons coconut oil
- 2 onions, chopped finely
- 1 (1-inch) piece fresh ginger, minced
- 3 garlic cloves, minced
- ½ teaspoon ground turmeric
- 2 ½ pound lamb shoulder, trimmed and cubed into 3-inch size
- Salt
- ground black pepper
- ½ teaspoon saffron threads, crumbled
- 1 cinnamon stick
- 3 cups of water
- 1 cup prunes, pitted and halved

Directions:

1. In a big pan, melt coconut oil on medium heat. Add onions, ginger, garlic cloves, and turmeric and sauté for about 3-5 minutes. Flavor the lamb with salt plus black pepper evenly.
2. In the pan, add lamb and saffron threads and cook for approximately 4-5 minutes. Add cinnamon stick and water and produce to some boil on high heat.
3. Adjust to low and simmer, covered for around 1½-120 minutes or till the desired doneness of lamb. Stir in prunes and simmer for approximately 20-a half-hour. Remove cinnamon stick and serve hot.

Nutrition:
Calories 393
Fat 12g
Carbs 10g
Protein 36g
Phosphorus 133.3mg
Potassium 0.16mg
Sodium 78mg

Roast Beef

Preparation Time: 25 minutes
Cooking Time: 55 minutes
Servings: 3
Ingredients:

- Quality rump or sirloin tip roast
- Pepper & herbs

Directions:

1. Place in a roasting pan on a shallow rack. Season with pepper and herbs. Insert meat thermometer in the center or thickest part of the roast.

2. Roast to the desired degree of doneness. After removing from over for about 15 minutes, let it chill. In the end, the roast should be moister than well done.

Nutrition:
Calories 158
Protein 24g
Fat 6g
Carbs 0g
Phosphorus 20 mg
Potassium 328mg
Sodium 55mg

CHAPTER 15:

Poultry

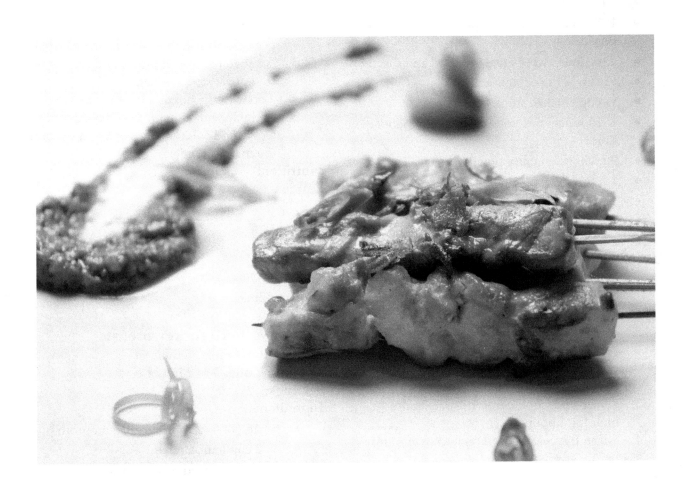

Chicken curry
Preparation Time: 10 minutes
Cooking Time: 4 minutes
Servings: 4
Ingredients

- 1lb skinless chicken breasts
- 1 medium onion, thinly sliced
- 1 15 ounce can chickpeas, drained and rinsed well
- 2 medium sweet squash, peeled and diced
- ½ cup light coconut milk
- ½ cup chicken stock (see recipe)
- 1 15ounce can sodium-free red pepper sauce
- 2 tablespoon curry powder
- 1 teaspoon low-sodium salt
- ½ cayenne powder
- 1 cup green peas
- 2 tablespoon lemon juice

Directions

1. Place the chicken breasts, onion, chickpeas, and sweet squash into a 4 to 6-quart slow cooker.
2. Mix the coconut milk, chicken stock, red pepper sauce, curry powder, salt, and cayenne together and pour into the slow cooker, stirring to coat well.
3. Cover and cook on low for 8 hours or high for 4 hours.
4. Stir in the peas and lemon juice 5 minutes before serving.

Nutrition:
Calories 302 Fat 5g
Carbs 43g Protein 24g
Fiber 9g Potassium 573mg Sodium 800mg

Apple & cinnamon spiced honey pork loin
Preparation Time: 20 minutes
Cooking Time: 6 hours
Servings: 6
Ingredients

- 1 2-3lb boneless pork loin roast
- ½ teaspoon low-sodium salt
- ¼ teaspoon pepper
- 1 tablespoon canola oil
- 3 medium apples, peeled and sliced
- ¼ cup honey
- 1 small red onion, halved and sliced
- 1 tablespoon ground cinnamon

Directions

1. Season the pork with salt and pepper.
2. Heat the oil in a skillet and brown the pork on all sides.
3. Arrange half the apples in the base of a 4 to 6-quart slow cooker.
4. Top with the honey and remaining apples.
5. Sprinkle with cinnamon and cover.
6. Cover and cook on low for 6-8 hours until the meat is tender.

Nutrition:
Calories 290
Fat 10g
Carbs 19g
Protein 29g
Fiber 2g
Potassium 789mg
Sodium 22mg

Lemon & herb turkey breasts
Preparation Time: 25 minutes
Cooking Time: 3 1/2 hours
Servings: 12
Ingredients

- 1 can (14-1/2 ounces) chicken broth
- 1/2 cup lemon juice
- 1/4 cup packed brown sugar
- 1/4 cup fresh sage
- 1/4 cup fresh thyme leaves
- 1/4 cup lime juice
- 1/4 cup cider vinegar
- 1/4 cup caper oil
- 1 envelope low-sodium onion soup mix
- 2 tablespoon Dijon mustard
- 1 tablespoon fresh marjoram, minced
- 1 teaspoon paprika
- 1 teaspoon garlic powder
- 1 teaspoon pepper
- ½ teaspoon low-sodium salt

- 2 2lb boneless skinless turkey breast halves

Directions

1. Make a marinade by blending all the ingredients in a blender.
2. Pour over the turkey and leave overnight.
3. Place the turkey and marinade in a 4 to 6-quart slow cooker and cover.
4. Cover and cook on high for 3-1/2 to 4-1/2 hours or until a thermometer reads 165°.

Nutrition:

Calories 219,
Fat 5g
Carbs 3g
Protein 36g
Fiber 0g
Potassium 576mg
Sodium 484mg

Beef chimichangas

Preparation Time: 10minutes
Cooking Time: 10-12 hours
Servings: 16
Ingredients

- Shredded beef
- 3lb boneless beef chuck roast, fat trimmed away
- 3 tablespoon low-sodium taco seasoning mix
- 1 10ounce canned low-sodium diced red peppers
- 6ounce canned diced green chilies with the juice
- 3 garlic cloves, minced
- To serve
- 16 medium flour tortillas
- Sodium-free refried beans
- Mexican rice, sour cream, cheddar cheese
- Guacamole, salsa, lettuce

Directions

1. Arrange the beef in a 5-quart or larger slow cooker.
2. Sprinkle over taco seasoning and coat well.
3. Add red peppers and garlic and cover.

4. Cook on low for 10 to 12 hours.
5. When cooked remove the beef and shred.
6. Make burritos out of the shredded beef, refried beans, Mexican rice, and cheese.
7. Bake for 10 minutes at 350° f until brown.
8. Serve with salsa, lettuce, and guacamole.

Nutrition:

Calories 249
Fat 18g
Carbs 3g
Protein 33g
Fiber 5g
Potassium 633mg
Sodium 457mg

Crockpot peachy pork chops

Preparation Time: 30minutes
Cooking Time: 2-3 hours
Servings: 8
Ingredients

- 4 large peaches, pitted and peeled
- 1 onion, finely minced
- ¼ cup ketchup
- ¼ cup low-sodium honey barbecue sauce
- 2 tablespoon brown sugar
- 1 tablespoon low sodium soy sauce
- ¼ teaspoon low-sodium garlic salt
- ½ teaspoon ground ginger
- 2lb boneless pork chops
- 3 tablespoon caper oil

Directions

1. Puree the peaches with a blender.
2. Mix the peach puree with the onion, ketchup, barbecue sauce, brown sugar, soy sauce, salt, garlic salt, and ginger.
3. Brown the pork chops in a large skillet then transfer to a 6-quart or larger slow cooker.
4. Pour the sauce over the pork chops and cover.
5. Cook for 5 to 6 hours on high.

Nutrition:

Calories 252 Fat 8g Carbs 18g
Protein 26g Fiber 1g Potassium 710mg
Sodium 325mg

Chicken salad balsamic
Preparation time: 15 minutes
Cooking Time: 15 minutes
Servings: 6
Ingredients

- 3 cup diced cold, cooked chicken
- 1 cup diced apple
- 1/2 cup diced celery
- 2 green onions, chopped
- 1/2 cup chopped walnuts
- 3 tablespoons. Balsamic vinegar
- 5 tablespoons. Caper oil
- Salt and pepper to taste

Directions

1. Toss together the celery, chicken, onion, walnuts, and apple in a big bowl.
2. Whisk the oil together with the vinegar in a small bowl. Pour the dressing over the salad. Then add pepper and salt to taste. Combine the ingredients thoroughly. Leave the mixture for 10-15 minutes. Toss once more and chill.

Nutrition:
Calories 336 Fat 26.8g
Carbs 6g
Protein 19gSodium 58 mg

Chicken salad with apples, grapes, and walnuts
Preparation Time: 25 minutes
Cooking Time: 25 minutes
Servings: 12
Ingredients

- 4 cooked chicken breasts, shredded
- 2 granny smith apples, cut into small chunks
- 2cupchopped walnuts, or to taste
- 1/2 red onion, chopped
- 3 stalks celery, chopped
- 3 tablespoons. Lemon juice
- 1/2cupvanilla yogurt
- 5 tablespoons. Creamy salad dressing (such as miracle whip®)
- 5 tablespoons. Mayonnaise
- 25 seedless red grapes, halved

Directions

1. In a big bowl, toss together the shredded chicken, lemon juice, apple chunks, celery, red onion, and walnuts.
2. Get another bowl and whisk together the dressing, vanilla yogurt, and mayonnaise. Pour over the chicken mixture. Toss to coat. Fold the grapes carefully into the salad.

Nutrition:
Calories 307
Fat 22.7g
Carbs 10.8g
Protein 17.3g
Sodium 128mg
Phosphorous 288mg
Potassium 334mg

Chicken strawberry spinach salad with ginger-lime dressing
Preparation Time: 10 minutes
Cooking Time: 30 minutes
Servings: 2
Ingredients

- 2 teaspoons. Corn oil
- 1 skinless, boneless chicken breast half - cut into bite-size pieces
- 1/2 teaspoon garlic powder
- 1 1/2 tablespoons. Mayonnaise
- 1/2 lime, juiced
- 1/2 teaspoon ground ginger
- 2 teaspoons. Milk
- 2cupfresh spinach, stems removed
- 4 fresh strawberries, sliced
- 1 1/2 tablespoons. Slivered almonds
- Freshly ground black pepper to taste

Directions

1. In a skillet, heat oil over medium heat. Add the chicken breast and garlic powder. Cook the chicken for 10 minutes per side. When the juices run clear, remove from heat and set aside.
2. Combine the lime juice, milk, mayonnaise, and ginger in a bowl.
3. Place the spinach on serving dishes. Top with strawberries and chicken. Then

sprinkle with almonds. Drizzle the salad with the dressing. Add pepper and serve.

Nutrition:
Calories 242
Fat 17.3g
Carbs 7.5g
Protein 15.8g
Sodium 117mg
Phosphorous 288mg
Potassium 334mg

Asian chicken satay
Preparation Time: 15 minutes
Cooking Time: 10 minutes
Servings: 6
Ingredients
- Juice of 2 limes
- Brown sugar – 2 tablespoons
- Minced garlic – 1 tablespoon
- Ground cumin – 2 teaspoons
- Boneless, skinless chicken breast – 12, cut into strips

Directions
1. In a bowl, stir together the cumin, garlic, brown sugar, and lime juice.
2. Add the chicken strips to the bowl and marinate in the refrigerator for 1 hour.
3. Heat the barbecue to medium-high.
4. Remove the chicken from the marinade and thread each strip onto wooden skewers that have been soaked in the water.
5. Grill the chicken for about 4 minutes per side or until the meat is cooked through but still juicy.

Nutrition:
Calories 78
Carbs 4g
Phosphorus 116mg
Potassium 108mg
Sodium 100mg
Protein 12g

Zucchini and turkey burger with jalapeno peppers
Preparation Time: 15 minutes
Cooking Time: 10 minutes
Servings: 4
Ingredients
- Turkey meat (ground) – 1 pound
- Zucchini (shredded) – 1 cup
- Onion (minced) – ½ cup
- Jalapeño pepper (seeded and minced) – 1
- Egg – 1
- Extra-spicy blend – 1 teaspoon
- Fresh polao peppers (seeded and sliced in half lengthwise)
- Mustard – 1 teaspoon

Directions
1. Start by taking a mixing bowl and adding in the turkey meat, zucchini, onion, jalapeño pepper, egg, and extra-spicy blend. Mix well to combine.
2. Divide the mixture into 4 equal portions. Form burger patties out of the same.
3. Prepare an electric griddle or an outdoor grill. Place the burger patties on the grill and cook until the top is blistered and tender. Place the sliced poblano peppers on the grill alongside the patties. Grilling the patties should take about 5 minutes on each side.
4. Once done, place the patties onto the buns and top them with grilled peppers.

Nutrition:
Calories 325 Protein 25g
Carbs 5g Fat 10g Sodium 128mg
Potassium 475mg Phosphorus 280mg
Fiber 1.6g

Gnocchi and chicken dumplings
Preparation Time: 10 minutes
Cooking Time: 40 minutes
Servings: 10
Ingredients
- Chicken breast – 2 pounds
- Gnocchi – 1 pound
- Light caper oil – ¼ cup

- Better than bouillon® chicken base – 1 tablespoon
- Chicken stock (reduced-sodium) – 6 cups
- Fresh celery (diced finely) – ½ cup
- Fresh onions (diced finely) – ½ cup
- Fresh carrots (diced finely) – ½ cup
- Fresh parsley (chopped) – ¼ cup
- Black pepper – 1 teaspoon
- Italian seasoning – 1 teaspoon

Directions

1. Start by placing the stock over a high flame. Add in the oil and let it heat through.
2. Add the chicken to the hot oil and shallow-fry until all sides turn golden brown.
3. Toss in the carrots, onions, and celery and cook for about 5 minutes. Pour in the chicken stock and let it cool on a high flame for about 30 minutes.
4. Reduce the flame and add in the chicken bouillon, Italian seasoning, and black pepper. Stir well.
5. Toss in the store-bought gnocchi and let it cook for about 15 minutes. Keep stirring.
6. Once done, transfer into a serving bowl. Add parsley and serve hot!

Nutrition:
Calories 196 Protein 28g
Carbs 38g Fat 10g
Sodium 121mg
Potassium 485mg
Fiber 2g

Creamy Turkey

Preparation Time: 12 minutes
Cooking Time: 10 minutes
Servings: 4
Ingredients:

- 4 skinless, boneless turkey breast halves
- Salt and pepper to taste
- ½ teaspoon ground black pepper
- ½ teaspoon garlic powder
- 1 (10.75 ounces) can chicken soup

Directions:

1. Preheat oven to 375 degrees F.
2. Clean turkey breasts and season with salt, pepper and garlic powder (or whichever seasonings you prefer) on both sides of turkey pieces.
3. Bake for 25 minutes, then add chicken soup and bake for 10 more minutes (or until done). Serve over rice or egg noodles.

Nutrition:
Calories 160, Sodium 157mg
Fibers 0.4g Carbs 0.4g Protein 25.6g
Potassium 152mg Phosphorus 85mg

Lemon Pepper Chicken Legs

Preparation Time: 5 minutes
Cooking Time: 25 minutes
Servings: 4
Ingredients:

- ½ tsp. garlic powder
- 2 tsp. baking powder
- 8 chicken legs
- 4 tbsp. salted butter, melted
- 1 tbsp. lemon pepper seasoning

Directions:

1. In a small container add the garlic powder and baking powder, then use this mixture to coat the chicken legs. Lay the chicken in the basket of your fryer.
2. Cook the chicken legs at 375°F for twenty-five minutes. Halfway through, turn them over and allow to cook on the other side.
3. When the chicken has turned golden brown, test with a thermometer to ensure it has reached an ideal temperature of 165°F. Remove from the fryer.
4. Mix together the melted butter and lemon pepper seasoning and toss with the chicken legs until the chicken is coated all over. Serve hot.

Nutrition:
Calories 132 Fat 16 g
Carbs 20 g   Protein 48 g
Phosphorous 132mg   Potassium 127mg
Sodium 121mg

Turkey Broccoli Salad

Preparation Time: 10 minutes
Cooking Time: 0 minutes
Servings: 4
Ingredients:

- 8 cups broccoli florets
- 3 cooked skinless, boneless chicken breast halves, cubed
- 6 green onions, chopped
- 1 cup mayonnaise
- ¼ cup apple cider vinegar
- ¼ cup honey

Directions:

1. Combine broccoli, chicken and green onions in a large bowl.
2. Whisk mayonnaise, vinegar, and honey together in a bowl until well blended.
3. Pour mayonnaise dressing over broccoli mixture; toss to coat.
4. Cover and refrigerate until chilled, if desired. Serve

Nutrition:
Calories 133
Sodium 23mg
Fibers 1.6g
Carbs 7.7g
Protein 6.2g
Potassium 157mg
Phosphorus 148 mg

Fruity Chicken Salad

Preparation Time: 10 minutes
Cooking Time: 5 minutes
Servings: 3
Ingredients:

- 4 skinless, boneless chicken breast halves - cooked and diced
- 1 stalk celery, diced
- 4 green onions, chopped
- 1 Golden Delicious apple - peeled, cored and diced
- 1/3 cup seedless green grapes, halved
- 1/8 teaspoon ground black pepper
- 3/4 cup light mayonnaise

Directions:

1. In a large container, add the celery, chicken, onion, apple, grapes, pepper, and mayonnaise.
2. Mix all together. Serve!

Nutrition:
Calories 196
Sodium 181mg
Carbs 15.6g
Fibers 1.2g
Protein 13.2g,
Sodium 123mg
Potassium 115mg
Phosphorus 88 mg

Buckwheat Salad

Preparation Time: 12 minutes
Cooking Time: 20 minutes
Servings: 3
Ingredients:

- 2 cups water
- 1 clove garlic, smashed
- 1 cup uncooked buckwheat
- 2 large cooked chicken breasts - cut into bite-size pieces
- 1 large red onion, diced
- 1 large green bell pepper, diced
- 1/4 cup chopped fresh parsley
- 1/4 cup chopped fresh chives
- 1/2 teaspoon salt
- 2/3 cup fresh lemon juice
- 1 tablespoon balsamic vinegar
- 1/4 cup caper oil

Directions:

1. Bring the water, garlic to a boil in a saucepan. Stir in the buckwheat, reduce heat to medium-low, cover, and simmer until the buckwheat is tender and the water has been absorbed, 15 to 20 minutes.
2. Discard the garlic clove and scrape the buckwheat into a large bowl.
3. Gently stir the chicken, onion, bell pepper, parsley, chives, and salt into the buckwheat.

4. Sprinkle with the caper oil, balsamic vinegar, and lemon juice. Stir until evenly mixed.

Nutrition:
Calories 199
Fat 8.3g
Sodium 108mg
Fiber 2.9g
Carbs 2g
Protein 13.6g
Potassium 262mg
Phosphorus 188 mg

Parmesan and Basil turkey Salad

Preparation Time: 15 minutes
Cooking Time: 35 minutes
Servings: 4
Ingredients:

- 2 whole skinless, boneless turkey breasts
- salt and pepper to taste
- 1 cup mayonnaise
- 1 cup chopped fresh basil
- 2 cloves crushed garlic
- 3 stalks celery, chopped
- 2/3 cup grated Parmesan cheese

Directions:

1. Season turkey with salt and pepper. Roast at 375 degrees F for 35 minutes, or until juices run clear. Let cool, and chop into chunks.
2. In a food processor, puree the mayonnaise, basil, garlic, and celery.
3. Combine the chunked turkey, pureed mixture, and Parmesan cheese; toss.
4. Refrigerate, and serve.

Nutrition:
Calories 303
Sodium 190mg
Fiber 0.4g
Carbs 4.7g
Protein 8.5g
Potassium 121mg
Phosphorus 100 mg

Cherry Chicken Salad

Preparation Time: 15 minutes
Cooking Time: 0 minutes
Servings: 4
Ingredients:

- 3 cooked, boneless chicken breast halves, diced
- 1/3 cup dried cherries
- 1/3 cup diced celery
- 1/3 cup low-fat mayonnaise
- 1/2 teaspoon ground black pepper
- 1/3 cup cubed apples (optional)

Directions:

1. In a large bowl, combine the chicken, dried cherries, celery, mayonnaise, and pepper and apple if desired.
2. Toss together well and refrigerate until chilled.
3. Serve on toasted cracked wheat bread

Nutrition:
Calories 281
Fat 11.8g
Sodium 586mg
Fiber 1.4g
Protein 14.7g
Potassium 55mg
Phosphorus 20 mg

Elegant Brunch Chicken Salad

Preparation Time: 20 minutes
Cooking Time: 10 minutes
Servings: 4
Ingredients:

- 1-pound skinless, boneless chicken breast halves
- 1 egg
- 1/4 teaspoon dry mustard
- 2 teaspoons hot water
- 1 tablespoon white wine vinegar
- 1 cup caper oil
- 2 cups halved seedless red grapes

Directions:

1. Boil water in a large pot. Add the chicken and simmer until cooked thoroughly approximately 10

minutes. Drain, cool and cut into cubes.

2. While boiling chicken, make the mayonnaise: Using a blender or hand-held electric mixer, beat the egg, mustard, water and vinegar until light and frothy.

3. Add the oil a tablespoon at a time, beating thoroughly after each addition. As the combination starts to thicken, you can add oil more quickly.

4. Continue until the mixture reaches the consistency of creamy mayonnaise.

5. In a large bowl, toss together the chicken, grapes and 1 cup of the mayonnaise. Stir until evenly coated, adding more mayonnaise if necessary. Refrigerate until serving.

Nutrition:
Calories 676
Sodium 56mg
Carbs 14.7g
Fiber 1.4g
Protein 28.1g
Potassium 183mg
Phosphorus 120 mg

Oven-Baked Turkey Thighs
Preparation Time: 10 minutes
Cooking Time: 30 minutes
Servings: 4
Ingredients:
- 10 ounces turkey thighs, skin on, bone-in
- 1/3 cup white wine
- 1 lemon
- 1 tablespoon fresh oregano
- 1/4 teaspoon cracked black pepper
- 1 tablespoon caper oil

Directions:
1. Heat the oven to 350 degrees F.
2. Add turkey thighs and white wine to an oven-proof pan. Squeeze half the lemon over turkey. Slice remaining

lemon and top turkey with lemon slices.

3. Season turkey with fresh oregano, cracked pepper and caper oil.

4. Bake turkey for 25 to 30 minutes or until internal temperature reaches 165 degrees F to 175 degrees F.

Nutrition:
Calories 189 Sodium 62mg
Fibers 0.9g Carbs 0.6g
Protein 20.8g
Potassium 232mg
Phosphorus 180mg

Southern Fried Chicken
Preparation Time: 5 minutes
Cooking Time: 26 minutes
Servings: 2
Ingredients:
- 2 x 6-oz. boneless skinless chicken breasts
- 2 tbsp. hot sauce
- ½ tsp. onion powder
- 1 tbsp. chili powder
- 2 oz. pork rinds, finely ground

Directions:
1. Chop the chicken breasts in half lengthways and rub in the hot sauce. Combine the onion powder with the chili powder, then rub into the chicken. Leave to marinate for at least a half hour.

2. Use the ground pork rinds to coat the chicken breasts in the ground pork rinds, covering them thoroughly. Place the chicken in your fryer.

3. Set the fryer at 350°F and cook the chicken for 13 minutes. Turn over the chicken and cook the other side for another 13 minutes or until golden.

4. Test the chicken with a meat thermometer. When fully cooked, it should reach 165°F. Serve hot, with the sides of your choice.

Nutrition:
Calories 408 Fat 19 g Carbs 10 g
Protein 35 gPhosphorous 216mg
Potassium 137mg
Sodium 153 mg

Cilantro Drumsticks
Preparation Time: 12 minutes
Cooking Time: 18 minutes
Servings: 4
Ingredients:

- 8 chicken drumsticks
- ½ cup chimichurri sauce
- ¼ cup lemon juice

Directions:
1. Coat the chicken drumsticks with chimichurri sauce and refrigerate in an airtight container for no less than an hour, ideally overnight.
2. When it's time to cook, pre-heat your fryer to 400°F.
3. Remove the chicken from refrigerator and allow return to room temperature for roughly twenty minutes.
4. Cook for eighteen minutes in the fryer. Drizzle with lemon juice to taste and enjoy.

Nutrition:
Calories 483
Fat 29 g
Carbs 16 g
Protein 36 g
Phosphorous 146mg
Potassium 227mg
Sodium 121 mg

Basil Chicken over Macaroni
Preparation Time: 10 minutes
Cooking Time: 30 minutes
Servings: 4
Ingredients:

- 1 (8 ounces) package macaroni
- 2 teaspoons caper oil
- 1/2 cup finely chopped onion
- 1 clove garlic, chopped
- 2 cups boneless chicken breast halves, cooked and cubed
- 1/4 cup chopped fresh basil
- 1/4 cup Parmesan cheese
- 1/2 teaspoon black pepper

Directions:
1. In a large pot of boiling water, cook macaroni until it is al dente, about 8 to 10 minutes. Drain, and set aside.
2. In a large skillet, heat oil over medium-high heat. Sauté the onions and garlic. Stir in the chicken, basil, and pepper.
3. Reduce heat to medium, and cover skillet. Simmer for about 5 minutes, stirring frequently,
4. Toss sauce with hot cooked macaroni to coat. Serve with Parmesan cheese.

Nutrition:
Calories 349
Sodium 65mg
Fiber 2.2g
Carbs 2.1g
Protein 28.5g
Potassium 286mg
Phosphorus 280 mg

Chicken Sauté
Preparation Time: 10 minutes
Cooking Time: 25 minutes
Servings: 2
Ingredients:

- 4 oz. chicken fillet
- 4 red peppers, peeled
- 1 bell pepper, chopped
- 1 teaspoon caper oil
- 1 cup of water
- 1 teaspoon salt
- 1 chili pepper, chopped
- ½ teaspoon saffron

Directions:
1. Pour water in the pan and bring it to boil.
2. Meanwhile, chop the chicken fillet.
3. Add the chicken fillet in the boiling water and cook it for 10 minutes or until the chicken is tender.
4. After this, put the chopped bell pepper and chili pepper in the skillet.
5. Add caper oil and roast the vegetables for 3 minutes.

6. Add chopped red peppers and mix up well.
7. Cook the vegetables for 2 minutes more.
8. Then add salt and a ¾ cup of water from chicken.
9. Add chopped chicken fillet and mix up.
10. Cook the sauté for 10 minutes over the medium heat.

Nutrition:
Calories 192
Fat 7.2 g
Fiber 3.8 g
Carbs 14.4 g
Protein 19.2 g
Phosphorous 216mg
Potassium 227mg
Sodium 101 mg

Grilled Marinated Chicken
Preparation Time: 35 minutes
Cooking Time: 20 minutes
Servings: 6
Ingredients:
- 2-pound chicken breast, skinless, boneless
- 2 tablespoons lemon juice
- 1 teaspoon sage
- ½ teaspoon ground nutmeg
- ½ teaspoon dried oregano
- 1 teaspoon paprika
- 1 teaspoon onion powder
- 2 tablespoons caper oil
- 1 teaspoon chili flakes
- 1 teaspoon salt
- 1 teaspoon apple cider vinegar

Directions:
1. Make the marinade: whisk together apple cider vinegar, salt, chili flakes, caper oil, onion powder, paprika, dried oregano, ground nutmeg, sage, and lemon juice.
2. Then rub the chicken with marinade carefully and leave for 25 minutes to marinate.
3. Meanwhile, preheat grill to 385F.
4. Place the marinated chicken breast in the grill and cook it for 10 minutes from each side.

5. Cut the cooked chicken on the servings.

Nutrition:
Calories 218
Fat 8.2 g
Fiber 0.8 g
Carbs 0.4 g
Protein 32.2 g
Calcium 29mg
Phosphorous 116mg
Potassium 207mg
Sodium 121 mg

Tasty Turkey Patties
Preparation Time: 10 minutes
Cooking Time: 12 minutes
Servings: 4
Ingredients:
- 14.5-ounces turkey
- 1-ounce cream cheese
- 1 large egg
- 1/8 teaspoon ground sage
- 1/2 teaspoon garlic powder
- 1/2 teaspoon black pepper
- 1 teaspoon onion powder
- 1 teaspoon Italian seasoning
- 3/4 cup graham crackers crumbs
- 3 tablespoons caper oil

Directions:
1. Set cream cheese out to soften.
2. Using a fork, mash turkey with juices in a medium bowl.
3. Add the cream cheese, egg, sage, garlic powder, black pepper, onion powder, Italian seasoning and graham crackers crumbs; mix well.
4. Form 4 patties.
5. Heat caper oil on low hotness, in a small skillet.
6. Fry patties for 5- to 6 minutes on each side or until crispy on the outside and heated thoroughly.

Nutrition:
Calories 270, Sodium 204mg
Fiber 1.1g Carbs 3.5g Protein 13.5g
Potassium 143mg Phosphorus 100 mg

CHAPTER 16:

Desserts

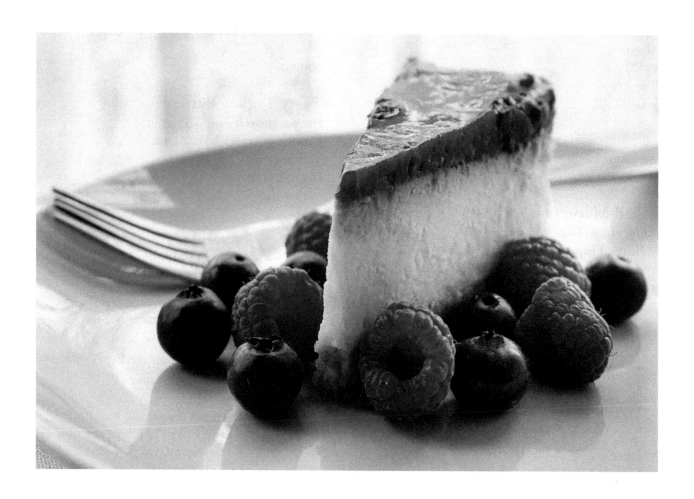

Baked Apples with Cherries and Walnuts

Preparation Time: 10 minutes
Cooking Time: 35 to 40 minutes
Servings: 6
Ingredients:

- 1/3 cup dried cherries, coarsely chopped
- 3 tablespoons chopped walnuts
- 1 tablespoon ground flaxseed meal
- 1 tablespoon firmly packed brown sugar
- 1 teaspoon ground cinnamon
- 1/8 teaspoon nutmeg
- 6 Golden Delicious apples, about 2 pounds total weight, washed and unpeeled
- 1/2 cup 100 percent apple juice
- 1/4 cup water
- 2 tablespoons dark honey
- 2 teaspoons extra-virgin caper oil

Directions:

1. Preheat the oven to 350°F.
2. In a small bowl, toss together the cherries, walnuts, flaxseed meal, brown sugar, cinnamon, and nutmeg until all the ingredients are evenly distributed. Set aside.
3. Working from the stem end, core each apple, stopping ¾ of an inch from the bottom.
4. Gently press the cherries into each apple cavity. Arrange the apples upright in a heavy ovenproof skillet or baking dish just large enough to hold them.
5. Pour the apple juice and water into the pan.
6. Drizzle the honey and oil evenly over the apples, and cover the pan snugly with aluminum foil. Bake until the apples are tender when pierced with a knife, 35 to 40 minutes.
7. Transfer the apples to individual plates and drizzle with the pan juices. Serve warm.

Nutrition:
Calories 162 Fat 5g Sodium 4mg
Potassium 148mg Carbs 30g Fiber 4g Protein 1g

Easy Peach Crumble

Preparation Time: 10 minutes
Cooking Time: 30 minutes
Servings: 8
Ingredients:

- 8 ripe peaches, peeled, pitted and sliced
- 3 tablespoons freshly squeezed lemon juice
- 1/2 teaspoon ground cinnamon
- 1/4 teaspoon ground nutmeg
- 1/2 cup oat flour
- 1/4 cup packed dark brown sugar
- 2 tablespoons margarine, cut into thin slices
- 1/4 cup quick-cooking oats

Directions:

1. Preheat the oven to 375°F. Lightly coat a 9-inch pie pan with cooking spray. Arrange peach slices in the prepared pie plate and sprinkle with the lemon juice, cinnamon, and nutmeg.
2. In a small bowl, whisk together the flour and brown sugar. With your fingers, crumble the margarine into the flour-sugar mixture. Add the uncooked oats and stir to mix. Sprinkle the flour mixture over the peaches.
3. Bake until the peaches are soft and the topping is browned, about 30 minutes.
4. Cut into 8 even slices and serve warm.

Nutrition:
Calories 130
Fat 4g
Sodium 42mg
Potassium 255mg
Carbs 28g
Fiber 3g
Protein: 2g

Lemon Thins

Preparation Time: 15 minutes
Cooking Time: 8 to 10 minutes
Servings: 30 cookies
Ingredients:

- Cooking spray
- 11/4 cups whole wheat pastry flour

- 1/3 cup cornstarch
- 1 1/2 teaspoons baking powder
- ¾ cup sugar, divided
- 2 tablespoons butter, softened
- 2 tablespoons extra-virgin caper oil
- 1 large egg white
- 3 teaspoons freshly grated lemon zest
- 1 1/2 teaspoons vanilla extract
- 4 tablespoons freshly squeezed lemon juice

Directions:

1. Preheat the oven to 350°F. Coat two baking sheets with cooking spray.
2. In a mixing bowl, whisk together the flour, cornstarch, and baking powder.
3. In another mixing bowl beat 1/2 cup of the sugar, the butter, and caper oil with an electric mixer on medium speed until fluffy.
4. Add the egg white, lemon zest, and vanilla and beat until smooth. Beat in the lemon juice.
5. Add the dry ingredients to the wet ingredients and fold in with a rubber spatula just until combined.

6. Drop the dough by the teaspoonful, 2 inches apart, onto the prepared baking sheets.
7. Place the remaining 1/4 cup sugar in a saucer. Coat the bottom of a wide-bottomed glass with cooking spray and dip it in the sugar. Flatten the dough with the glass bottom into 2 1/2-inch circles, dipping the glass in the sugar each time.
8. Bake the cookies until they are just starting to brown around the edges, 8 to 10 minutes. Transfer to a flat surface (not a rack) to crisp.

Nutrition: (1 cookie)
Calories 40 Fat 2g
Sodium 26mg
Potassium 3mg
Carbs 5g
Fiber 1g
Protein: 1g

Snickerdoodle Chickpea Blondies

Servings: 15
Preparation Time: 10 minutes
Cooking Time: 30 to 35 minutes
Ingredients:

- 1 (15-ounce) can chickpeas, drained and rinsed
- 3 tablespoons nut butter of choice
- ¾ teaspoon baking powder
- 2 teaspoons vanilla extract
- 1/8 teaspoon baking soda
- ¾ cup brown sugar
- 1 tablespoon unsweetened applesauce
- 1/4 cup ground flaxseed meal
- 2 1/4 teaspoons cinnamon

Directions:

1. Preheat the oven to 350°F. Grease an 8-by-8-inch baking pan.
2. Blend all ingredients in a food processor until very smooth. Scoop into the prepared baking pan.
3. Bake until the tops are medium golden brown, 30 to 35 minutes. Allow the brownies to cool completely before cutting.

Nutrition:
Calories 85
Fat 2g
Sodium 7mg
Potassium 62mg
Carbs 16g
Fiber 2g
Protein 3g

Chocolate Chia Seed Pudding

Preparation Time: 15 minutes, plus 3 to 5 hours or overnight to rest
Cooking Time: 0 minutes
Servings: 4
Ingredients:

- 1 1/2 cups unsweetened vanilla almond milk
- 1/4 cup unsweetened cocoa powder
- 1/4 cup maple syrup (or substitute any sweetener)
- 1/2 teaspoon vanilla extract

- 1/3 cup chia seeds
- 1/2 cup strawberries
- 1/4 cup blueberries
- 1/4 cup raspberries
- 2 tablespoons unsweetened coconut flakes
- 1/4 to 1/2 teaspoon ground cinnamon (optional)

Directions:

1. Add the almond milk, cocoa powder, maple syrup, and vanilla extract to a blender and blend until smooth. Whisk in chia seeds.
2. In a small bowl, gently mash the strawberries with a fork. Distribute the strawberry mash evenly to the bottom of 4 glass jars.
3. Pour equal portions of the blended milk-cocoa mixture into each of the jars and let the pudding rest in the refrigerator until it achieves a pudding like consistency, at least 3 to 5 hours and up to overnight.

Nutrition:
Calories 189
Fat 7g
Sodium 60mg
Potassium 232mg
Carbs 28g
Fiber 10g
Protein 6g

Chocolate-Mint Truffles

Preparation Time: 45 minutes
Cooking Time: 5 hours
Servings: 60 small truffles
Ingredients:

- 14 ounces semisweet chocolate, coarsely chopped
- ¾ cup half-and-half
- 1/2 teaspoon pure vanilla extract
- 11/2 teaspoon peppermint extract
- 2 tablespoons unsalted butter, softened
- ¾ cup naturally unsweetened or Dutch-process cocoa powder

Directions:

1. Place semisweet chocolate in a large heatproof bowl.
2. Microwave in four 15-second increments, stirring after each, for a total of 60 seconds. Stir until almost completely melted. Set aside.
3. In a small saucepan over medium heat, heat the half-and-half, whisking occasionally, until it just begins to boil. Remove from the heat, then whisk in the vanilla and peppermint extracts.
4. Pour the mixture over the chocolate and, using a wooden spoon, gently stir in one direction.
5. Once the chocolate and cream are smooth, stir in the butter until it is combined and melted.
6. Cover with plastic wrap pressed on the top of the mixture, and then let it sit at room temperature for 30 minutes.
7. After 30 minutes, place the mixture in the refrigerator until it is thick and can hold a ball shape, about 5 hours.
8. Line a large baking sheet with parchment paper or a use a silicone baking mat. Set aside.
9. Remove the mixture from the refrigerator. Place the cocoa powder in a bowl.
10. Scoop 1 teaspoon of the ganache and, using your hands, roll into a ball. Roll the ball in the cocoa powder, the place on the prepared baking sheet. (You can coat your palms with a little cocoa powder to prevent sticking).
11. Serve immediately or cover and store at room temperature for up to 1 week.

Nutrition:
Calories 21
Fat 2g
Sodium 2mg
Potassium 21mg
Carbs 2g
Fiber 1g
Protein 15g

Personal Mango Pies
Preparation Time: 15 minutes
Cooking Time: 14 to 16 minutes
Servings: 12
Ingredients:

- Cooking spray
- 12 small wonton wrappers
- 1 tablespoon cornstarch
- 1/2 cup water
- 3 cups finely chopped mango (fresh, or thawed from frozen, no sugar added)
- 2 tablespoons brown sugar (not packed)
- 1/2 teaspoon cinnamon
- 1 tablespoon light whipped butter or buttery spread

Directions:

1. Unsweetened coconut flakes (optional)
2. Preheat the oven to 350°F.
3. Spray a 12-cup muffin pan with nonstick cooking spray.
4. Place a wonton wrapper into each cup of the muffin pan, pressing it into the bottom and up along the sides.
5. Lightly spray the wrappers with nonstick spray. Bake until lightly browned, about 8 minutes.
6. Meanwhile, in a medium nonstick saucepan, combine the cornstarch with the water and stir to dissolve. Add the mango, brown sugar, and cinnamon and turn heat to medium.
7. Stirring frequently, cook until the mangoes have slightly softened and the mixture is thick and gooey, 6 to 8 minutes.
8. Remove the mango mixture from heat and stir in the butter.
9. Spoon the mango mixture into wonton cups, about 3 tablespoons each. Top with coconut flakes (if using) and serve warm.

Nutrition:
Calories 61 Fat 1g
Sodium 52mg
Potassium 77mg
Carbs 14g
Fiber 1g
Protein 1g

Grilled Peach Sundaes
Preparation Time: 15 minutes
Cooking Time: 5 minutes
Servings: 1
Ingredients:

- 1 tbsp. toasted unsweetened coconut
- 1 tsp. canola oil
- 2 peaches, halved and pitted
- 2 scoops non-fat vanilla yogurt, frozen

Directions:

1. Brush the peaches with oil and grill until tender.
2. Place peach halves on a bowl and top with frozen yogurt and coconut.

Nutrition:
Calories 61
Carbs 2g
Protein 2g
Fats 6g
Phosphorus 32mg
Potassium 85mg
Sodium 30mg

Blueberry Swirl Cake
Preparation Time: 15 minutes
Cooking Time: 45 minutes
Servings: 9
Ingredients:

- 1/2 cup margarine
- 1 1/4 cups reduced fat milk
- 1 cup granulated sugar
- 1 egg
- 1 egg white
- 1 tbsp. lemon zest, grated
- 1 tsp. cinnamon
- 1/3 cup light brown sugar
- 2 1/2 cups fresh blueberries
- 2 1/2 cups self-rising flour

Directions:

1. Cream the margarine and granulated sugar using an electric mixer at high speed until fluffy.
2. Add the egg and egg white and beat for another two minutes.

3. Add the lemon zest and reduce the speed to low.
4. Add the flour with milk alternately.
5. In a greased 13x19 pan, spread half of the batter and sprinkle with blueberry on top. Add the remaining batter.
6. Bake in a 350-degree Fahrenheit preheated oven for 45 minutes.
7. Let it cool on a wire rack before slicing and serving.

Nutrition:
Calories 384
Carbs 63g
Protein 7g
Fat 13g
Phosphorus 264mg
Potassium 158mg
Sodium 456mg

Peanut Butter Cookies
Preparation Time: 15 minutes
Cooking Time: 24 minutes
Servings: 24
Ingredients:
- 1/4 cup granulated sugar
- 1 cup unsalted peanut butter
- 1 tsp. baking soda
- 2 cups all-purpose flour
- 2 large eggs
- 2 tbsp. butter
- 2 tsp. pure vanilla extract
- 4 ounces softened cream cheese

Directions:
1. Line a cookie sheet with a non-stick liner. Set aside.
2. In a bowl, mix flour, sugar and baking soda. Set aside.
3. On a mixing bowl, combine the butter, cream cheese and peanut butter.
4. Mix on high speed until it forms a smooth consistency. Add the eggs and vanilla gradually while mixing until it forms a smooth consistency.

5. Add the almond flour mixture slowly and mix until well combined.
6. The dough is ready once it starts to stick together into a ball.
7. Scoop the dough using a 1 tablespoon cookie scoop and drop each cookie on the prepared cookie sheet.
8. Press the cookie with a fork and bake for 10 to 12 minutes at 350oF.

Nutrition:
Calories 138 Carbs 12g
Protein 4g Fat 9g
Phosphorus 60mg
Potassium 84mg
Sodium 31mg

Deliciously Good Scones
Preparation Time: 15 minutes
Cooking Time: 12 minutes
Servings: 10
Ingredients:
- 1/4 cup dried cranberries
- 1/4 cup sunflower seeds
- 1/2 teaspoon baking soda
- 1 large egg
- 2 cups all-purpose flour
- 2 tablespoon honey

Directions:
1. Preheat the oven to 3500F.
2. Grease a baking sheet. Set aside.
3. In a bowl, mix the salt, baking soda and flour. Add the dried fruits, nuts and seeds. Set aside.
4. In another bowl, mix the honey and eggs.
5. Add the wet ingredients to the dry ingredients. Use your hands to mix the dough.
6. Create 10 small round dough and place them on the baking sheet.
7. Bake for 12 minutes.

Nutrition:
Calories 44 Carbs 27g
Protein 4g Fat 3g
Phosphorus 59mg
Potassium 92mg Sodium 65mg

Mixed Berry Cobbler
Preparation Time: 15 minutes
Cooking Time: 4 hours
Servings: 8
Ingredients:

- 1/4 cup coconut milk
- 1/4 cup ghee
- 1/4 cup honey
- 1/2 cup almond flour
- 1/2 cup tapioca starch
- 1/2 tablespoon cinnamon
- 1/2 tablespoon coconut sugar
- 1 teaspoon vanilla
- 12 ounces frozen raspberries
- 16 ounces frozen wild blueberries
- 2 teaspoon baking powder
- 2 teaspoon tapioca starch

Directions:

1. Place the frozen berries in the slow cooker. Add honey and 2 teaspoons of tapioca starch. Mix to combine.
2. In a bowl, mix the tapioca starch, almond flour, coconut milk, ghee, baking powder and vanilla. Sweeten with sugar. Place this pastry mix on top of the berries.
3. Set the slow cooker for 4 hours.

Nutrition:
Calories: 146
Carbs 33g
Protein 1g
Fat 3g
Phosphorus 29mg
Potassium 133mg
Sodium 4mg

Blueberry Espresso Brownies
Preparation Time: 15 minutes
Cooking Time: 30 minutes
Servings: 12
Ingredients:

- 1/4 cup organic cocoa powder
- 1/4 teaspoon salt
- 1/2 cup raw honey
- 1/2 teaspoon baking soda
- 1 cup blueberries
- 1 cup coconut cream
- 1 tablespoon cinnamon
- 1 tablespoon ground coffee
- 2 teaspoon vanilla extract
- 3 eggs

Directions:

1. Preheat the oven to 3250F.
2. In a bow mix together coconut cream, honey, eggs, cinnamon, honey, vanilla, baking soda, coffee and salt.
3. Use a mixer to combine all ingredients.
4. Fold in the blueberries
5. Pour the batter in a greased baking dish and bake for 30 minutes or until a toothpick inserted in the middle comes out clean.
6. Remove from the oven and let it cool.

Nutrition:
Calories 168
Carbs 20g
Protein 4g
Fats 10g
Phosphorus 79mg
Potassium 169mg
Sodium 129mg

Coffee Brownies
Preparation Time: 15 minutes
Cooking Time: 20 minutes
Servings: 4
Ingredients:

- 3 eggs, beaten
- 2 tablespoons cocoa powder
- 2 teaspoons Erythritol
- 1/2 cup almond flour
- 1/2 cup organic almond milk

Directions:

1. Place the eggs in the mixing bowl and combine them with Erythritol and almond milk.
2. With the help of the hand mixer, whisk the liquid until homogenous.

3. Then add almond flour and cocoa powder.
4. Whisk the mixture until smooth.
5. Take the non-sticky brownie mold and transfer the cocoa mass inside it.
6. Flatten it gently with the help of the spatula. The flattened mass should be thin.
7. Preheat the oven to 365F.
8. Transfer the brownie in the oven and bake it for 20 minutes.
9. Then chill the cooked brownies at least till the room temperature and cut into serving bars.

Nutrition:
Calories 78
Fat 5.8g
Fiber 1.3g
Carbs 2.7g
Protein 5.5g
Sodium 123mg
Phosphorus 79mg
Potassium: 169mg

Fragrant Lava Cake
Preparation Time: 10 minutes
Cooking Time: 15 minutes
Servings: 5
Ingredients:

- 1 teaspoon baking powder
- 1 teaspoon vanilla extract
- 2 eggs, whisked
- 4 tablespoons cocoa powder
- 2 tablespoons Erythritol
- 8 tablespoons heavy cream
- 4 teaspoon almond flour
- Cooking spray

Directions:
1. Whisk the eggs together with heavy cream.
2. Then add vanilla extract, Erythritol, cocoa powder, and almond flour.
3. Mix the mixture until smooth.
4. Spray the mini cake molds with the cooking spray.
5. Preheat the oven to 350F.

6. Pour the cake mixture into the cake molds and place in the oven.
7. Bake the cakes for 15 minutes.
8. Then remove the lava cakes from the oven and discard from the cake molds.
9. Serve the lava cakes only hot.

Nutrition:
Calories 218 Fat 19.1g
Fiber 3.7g Carbs 8.3g
Protein 8.1g Phosphorus 79mg
Potassium 169mg

Almond Butter Mousse
Preparation Time: 7 minutes
Cooking Time: 7 minutes
Servings: 3
Ingredients:

- 2 strawberries
- 1 cup of coconut milk
- 1/2 teaspoon vanilla extract
- 2 teaspoon Erythritol
- 4 tablespoons almond butter
- ¾ teaspoon ground cinnamon

Directions:
1. Pour coconut milk in the food processor.
2. Add vanilla extract, Erythritol, almond butter, and ground cinnamon.
3. Blend the mixture until smooth.
4. Ten transfer it in the saucepan and start to preheat it over the medium heat.
5. Stir it all the time.
6. When the mousse starts to be thick, remove it from the heat and stir.
7. Pour the mousse into the serving glasses.
8. Slice the strawberries.
9. Top the mousse with the strawberries.

Nutrition:
Calories 321 Fat 31.1g
Fiber 4.4g Carbs 9.6g
Protein 6.4g Phosphorus 79mg
Potassium: 169mg

Almond Truffles

Preparation Time: 15 minutes
Cooking Time: 5 minutes
Servings: 5
Ingredients:

- 1/2 cup almond flour
- 2 teaspoons almond butter
- ¾ teaspoon ground cinnamon
- 1 teaspoon liquid stevia
- 1 oz. dark chocolate
- 1 tablespoon heavy cream

Directions:

1. Mix up together almond flour and almond butter.
2. Add ground cinnamon and liquid stevia.
3. Mix up the mixture until smooth.
4. Then make 5 truffles and place them on the baking paper.
5. Freeze them for 15 minutes in the freezer.
6. Meanwhile, preheat dark chocolate and heavy cream.
7. When the mixture is homogenous, the chocolate batter is cooked.
8. Remove the truffles from the freezer and sprinkle them with the chocolate batter.
9. Let the cooked truffles chill.

Nutrition:
Calories 98
Fat 8.1g
Fiber 1.5g
Carbs 5.4g
Protein 2.2g
Phosphorus 79mg
Potassium 169mg

Blueberry Cheesecake

Preparation Time: 20 minutes
Cooking Time: 55 minutes
Servings: 8
Ingredients:

- 2 tablespoons butter
- 1 teaspoon of cocoa powder
- 1/2 cup almond flour
- 2 cups cream cheese
- 1 tablespoon blueberry
- 2 tablespoons Erythritol
- 4 eggs, beaten
- 1 teaspoon vanilla extract

Directions:

1. Make the cheesecake crust: mix up together butter, cocoa powder, and almond flour and knead the dough.
2. Then place the dough into the 9-inch springform pan and flatten to get the shape of pie crust.
3. Freeze it in the freezer.
4. Meanwhile, blend the cream cheese until it is a soft and little bit fluffy.
5. Then add eggs, Erythritol, blueberries, and vanilla extract.
6. Blend the mixture until smooth.
7. Remove the pie crust from the freezer.
8. Put the cream cheese mixture over the pie crust and flatten it well.
9. Preheat the oven to 355F and place the cheesecake inside.
10. Cook the cheesecake for 55 minutes.
11. Then switch off the oven and let the cake sit for 25 minutes more. The perfect texture of the cheesecake will be reached after 7 hours of chilling.
12. Slice the cheesecake into the servings.

Nutrition:
Calories 272 Fat 26.2g
Fiber 0.3g Carbs 2.5g
Protein 7.6g
Phosphorus 79mg
Potassium 169mg

CHAPTER 17:

Sides

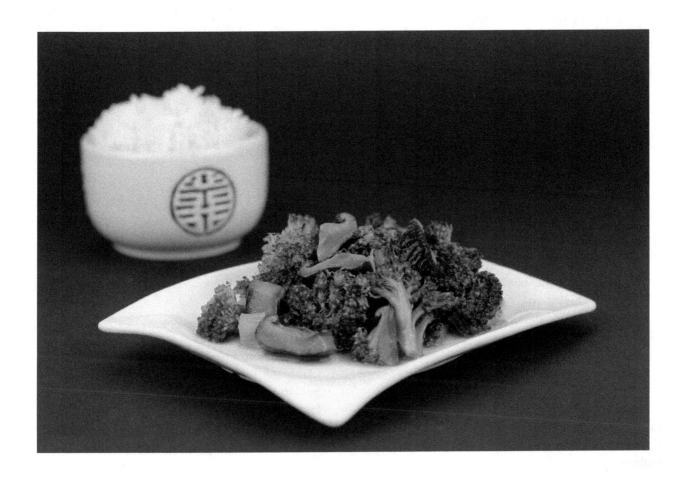

Ginger Cauliflower Rice
Preparation Time: 10 minutes
Cooking Time: 10 minutes
Servings: 4
Ingredients:

- 5 cups cauliflower florets
- 3 tablespoons coconut oil
- 4 ginger slices, grated
- 1 tablespoon coconut vinegar
- 3 garlic cloves, minced
- 1 tablespoon chives, minced
- A pinch of sea salt
- Black pepper to taste

Directions:

1. Put cauliflower florets in a food processor and pulse well.
2. Heat up a pan with the oil over medium-high heat, add ginger, stir and cook for 3 minutes.
3. Add cauliflower rice and garlic, stir and cook for 7 minutes.
4. Add salt, black pepper, vinegar, and chives, stir, cook for a few seconds more, divide between plates and serve.
5. Enjoy!

Nutrition:
Calories 125 Fat 10,4g
Fiber 3,2g Carbs 7,9g
Protein 2,7 Phosphorus 110mg
Potassium 117mg
Sodium 75mg

Basil Zucchini Spaghetti
Preparation Time: 1 hour and 10 minutes
Cooking Time: 10 minutes
Servings: 4
Ingredients:

- 1/3 cup coconut oil, melted
- 4 zucchinis, cut with a spiralizer
- ¼ cup basil, chopped
- A pinch of sea salt
- Black pepper to taste
- ½ cup walnuts, chopped
- 2 garlic cloves, minced

Directions:

2. In a bowl, mix zucchini spaghetti with salt and pepper, toss to coat, leave aside for 1 hour, drain well and put in a bowl.
3. Heat up a pan with the oil over medium-high heat, add zucchini spaghetti and garlic, stir and cook for 5 minutes.
4. Add basil and walnuts and black pepper, stir and cook for 3 minutes more.
5. Divide between plates and serve as a side dish
6. Enjoy!

Nutrition:
Calories 287
Fat 27,8g
Fiber 3,3g
Carbs 8,7g
Protein 6,3g
Phosphorus 110mg
Potassium 117mg
Sodium 75mg

Braised Cabbage
Preparation Time: 10 minutes
Cooking Time: 10 minutes
Servings: 4
Ingredients:

- 1 small cabbage head, shredded
- 2 tablespoons water
- A drizzle of caper oil
- 6 ounces shallots, cooked and chopped
- A pinch of black pepper
- A pinch of sweet paprika
- 1 tablespoon dill, chopped

Directions:

1. Heat up a pan with the oil over medium heat, add the cabbage and the water, stir and sauté for 5 minutes.
2. Add the rest of the ingredients, toss, cook for 5 minutes more, divide

everything between plates and serve as a side dish!

3. Enjoy!

Nutrition:
Calories 91
Fat 0,5g
Fiber 5,8g
Carbs 20,8g
Protein 4,1g
Phosphorus 120mg
Potassium 127mg
Sodium 75mg

Cauliflower and Leeks

Preparation Time: 10 minutes
Cooking Time: 20 minutes
Servings: 4
Ingredients:

- 1 and ½ cups leeks, chopped
- 1 and ½ cups cauliflower florets
- 2 garlic cloves, minced
- 1 and ½ cups artichoke hearts
- 2 tablespoons coconut oil, melted
- Black pepper to taste

Directions:

1. Heat up a pan with the oil over medium-high heat, add garlic, leeks, cauliflower florets and artichoke hearts, stir and cook for 20 minutes.
2. Add black pepper, stir, divide between plates and serve.
3. Enjoy!

Nutrition:
Calories 192
Fat 6,9g
Fiber 8,2g
Carbs 35,1g
Protein 5,1g
Phosphorus 110mg
Potassium 117mg
Sodium 75mg

Eggplant and Mushroom Sauté

Preparation Time: 10 minutes
Cooking Time: 30 minutes
Servings: 4
Ingredients:

- 2 pounds oyster mushrooms, chopped
- 6 ounces shallots, peeled, chopped
- 1 yellow onion, chopped
- 2 eggplants, cubed
- 3 celery stalks, chopped
- 1 tablespoon parsley, chopped
- A pinch of sea salt
- Black pepper to taste
- 1 tablespoon savory, dried
- 3 tablespoons coconut oil, melted

Directions:

1. Heat up a pan with the oil over medium high heat, add onion, stir and cook for 4 minutes.
2. Add shallots, stir and cook for 4 more minutes.
3. Add eggplant pieces, mushrooms, celery, savory and black pepper to taste, stir and cook for 15 minutes.
4. Add parsley, stir again, cook for a couple more minutes, divide between plates and serve.
5. Enjoy!

Nutrition:
Calories 1013 Fat 10,9g
Fiber 35,5 Carbs 156,5g
Protein 69,1g Phosphorus 210mg
Potassium 217mg
Sodium 105mg

Mint Zucchini

Preparation Time: 10 minutes
Cooking Time: 7 minutes
Servings: 4
Ingredients:

- 2 tablespoons mint
- 2 zucchinis, halved lengthwise and then slice into half moons
- 1 tablespoon coconut oil, melted

- ½ tablespoon dill, chopped
- A pinch of cayenne pepper

Directions:

1. Heat up a pan with the oil over medium-high heat, add zucchinis, stir and cook for 6 minutes.
2. Add cayenne, dill and mint, stir, cook for 1 minute more, divide between plates and serve.
3. Enjoy!

Nutrition:
Calories 46
Fat 3,6g
Fiber 1,3g
Carbs 3,5g
Protein 1,3g
Phosphorus 120mg
Potassium 127mg
Sodium 75mg

Celery and Kale Mix

Preparation Time: 10 minutes
Cooking Time: 20 minutes
Servings: 4
Ingredients:

- 2 celery stalks, chopped
- 5 cups kale, torn
- 1 small red bell pepper, chopped
- 3 tablespoons water
- 1 tablespoon coconut oil, melted

Directions:

1. Heat up a pan with the oil over medium-high heat, add celery, stir and cook for 10 minutes.
2. Add kale, water, and bell pepper, stir and cook for 10 minutes more.
3. Divide between plates and serve.
4. Enjoy!

Nutrition:
Calories 81 Fat 3,5g
Fiber 1,8g
Carbs 11,3g Protein 2,9g
Phosphorus 120mg
Potassium 147mg
Sodium 75mg

Kale, Mushrooms and Red Chard Mix

Preparation Time: 10 minutes
Cooking Time: 17 minutes
Servings: 4
Ingredients:

- ½ pound brown mushrooms, sliced
- 5 cups kale, roughly chopped
- 1 and ½ tablespoons coconut oil
- 3 cups red chard, chopped
- 2 tablespoons water
- Black pepper to taste

Directions:

1. Heat up a pan with the oil over medium high heat, add mushrooms, stir and cook for 5 minutes.
2. Add red chard, kale and water, stir and cook for 10 minutes.
3. Add black pepper to taste, stir and cook 2 minutes more.
4. Divide between plates and serve.
5. Enjoy!

Nutrition:
Calories 97g
Fat 3,4g
Fiber 2,3g
Carbs 13,3g
Protein 5,4g
Phosphorus 110mg
Potassium 117mg
Sodium 75mg

Bok Choy and Beets

Preparation Time: 10 minutes
Cooking Time: 30 minutes
Servings: 4
Ingredients:

- 1 tablespoon coconut oil
- 4 cups bok choy, chopped
- 3 beets, cut into quarters and thinly sliced
- 2 tablespoons water
- A pinch of cayenne pepper

Directions:

1. Put water in a large saucepan, add the beets, bring to a boil over medium

heat, cover, and cook for 20 minutes and drain.

2. Heat up a pan with the oil over medium high heat, add the bok choy and the water, stir and cook for 10 minutes.
3. Add beets and cayenne pepper, stir, cook for 2 minutes more, divide between plates and serve as a side dish!
4. Enjoy!

Nutrition:
Calories 71g
Fat 3,7g Fiber 2,2g
Carbs 9g Protein 2,3g
Phosphorus 110mg
Potassium 117mg
Sodium 75mg

Broccoli and Almonds Mix
Preparation Time: 10 minutes
Cooking Time: 11 minutes
Servings: 4
Ingredients:
- 1 tablespoon caper oil
- 1 garlic clove, minced
- 1-pound broccoli florets
- 1/3 cup almonds, chopped
- Black pepper to taste

Directions:
1. Heat up a pan with the oil over medium-high heat, add the almonds, stir, cook for 5 minutes and transfer to a bowl,
2. Heat up the same pan again over medium-high heat, add broccoli and garlic, stir, cover and cook for 6 minutes more.
3. Add the almonds and black pepper to taste, stir, divide between plates and serve.
4. Enjoy!

Nutrition:
Calories 116g Fat 7,8g Fiber 4g
Carbs 9,5g Protein 4,9g Phosphorus 110mg
Potassium 117mg
Sodium 75mg

Squash and Cranberries
Preparation Time: 10 minutes
Cooking Time: 30 minutes
Servings: 2
Ingredients:
- 1 tablespoon coconut oil
- 1 butternut squash, peeled and cubed
- 2 garlic cloves, minced
- 1 small yellow onion, chopped
- 12 ounces coconut milk
- 1 teaspoon curry powder
- 1 teaspoon cinnamon powder
- ½ cup cranberries

Directions:
1. Spread squash pieces on a lined baking sheet, place in the oven at 425 degrees F, bake for 15 minutes and leave to one side.
2. Heat up a pan with the oil over medium high heat, add garlic and onion, stir and cook for 5 minutes.
3. Add roasted squash, stir and cook for 3 minutes.
4. Add coconut milk, cranberries, cinnamon and curry powder, stir and cook for 5 minutes more.
5. Divide between plates and serve as a side dish!
6. Enjoy!

Nutrition:
Calories 518g
Fat 47,6g
Fiber 7,3g
Carbs 24,9
Protein 5,3g
Phosphorus 110mg
Potassium 117mg
Sodium 75mg

Creamy Chard
Preparation Time: 10 minutes
Cooking Time: 10 minutes
Servings: 2
Ingredients:
- Juice of ½ lemon
- 1 tablespoon coconut oil

- 12 ounces coconut milk
- 1 bunch chard
- A pinch of sea salt
- Black pepper to taste

Directions:

1. Heat up a pan with the oil over medium-high heat, add chard, stir and cook for 5 minutes.
2. Add lemon juice, a pinch of salt, black pepper, and coconut milk, stir and cook for 5 minutes more.
3. Divide between plates and serve as a side.
4. Enjoy!

Nutrition:

Calories 453
Fat 47,4g
Fiber 4g
Carbs 10,1g
Protein 4,2g
Phosphorus 130mg
Potassium 1127mg
Sodium 85mg

Conclusion

Managing chronic kidney disease (CKD) requires lifestyle adjustments, but it might help to know that you're not alone. Over 31 million people in the United States are diagnosed with some malfunction of their kidneys or are battling kidney disease. As a registered dietitian (RD) with extensive experience assisting patients in taking control over their kidney disease, I have helped patients not only manage the physical symptoms associated with this disease but also cope with the emotional toll that this life change can take. Without knowing what the future holds, uncertainty, fear, depression, and anxiety can be common. It may even feel like dialysis is inevitable, and you may be asking yourself if it is worth the time or effort to try and manage this stage of the disease or if it's even possible to delay the progression. As an expert in this field, I can assure you it is not just possible; it's yours to achieve—only 1 in 50 diagnosed with CKD end up on dialysis. So together, with the right tools, we can work to delay and ultimately prevent end-stage renal disease and dialysis. Success is earned through diet modifications and lifestyle changes. Using simple, manageable strategies, I have watched firsthand as my patients empowered themselves with knowledge. They have gone on to lead full, productive, and happy lives, continuing to work, play, and enjoy spending time with their loved ones—just the way it should be!

Only 1 in 50 diagnosed with CKD end up on dialysis. Diet is a vital part of treatment for CKD, and it can help immensely in slowing the progression of the disease. Some ingredients help the kidneys function, while others make the kidneys work harder. This book has focused on crowding out the unhealthy with healthy and helpful. Also, targeting factors like salt and carbohydrate intake are important to reduce the risk of hypertension, diabetes, and other diseases that can result from kidney failure. I can't emphasize enough the importance of consulting a dietitian throughout the progression of CKD to optimize health, and this book is a good start, as it's designed specifically for the treatment of this population.

In this time of change and uncertainty, the knowledge you gain from these pages will give you the power to take your life into your hands and make changes to benefit you in the short and long term. I hope to educate and inspire you with new, easy ways to change the trajectory of your health. Adopting a kidney-friendly lifestyle can be challenging at first, but following these recipes will reduce the anxiety associated with selecting smart food options for your everyday life. And lest you worry that your new diet is restrictive or unsustainable, I want to assure you that these recipes are both easy and delicious, and they will give you a realistic, satisfying way to make this lifestyle change. This book will guide you at each step of the way. In doing so, it will help take the stress of meal planning out of the equation and help you focus on the truly important things in life.

I hope you have learned something!

Appendix: Conversion Tables

Volume Equivalents (Liquid)

US STANDARD	US STANDARD (OUNCES)	METRIC (APPROXIMATE)
2 tablespoons	1 fl. oz.	30 mL
¼ cup	2 fl. oz.	60 mL
½ cup	4 fl. oz.	120 mL
1 cup	8 fl. oz.	240 mL
1½ cups	12 fl. oz.	355 mL
2 cups or 1 pint	16 fl. oz.	475 mL
4 cups or 1 quart	32 fl. oz.	1 L
1 gallon	128 fl. oz.	4 L

Volume Equivalents (Dry)

US STANDARD	METRIC (APPROXIMATE)
¼ teaspoon	1 mL
½ teaspoon	2 mL
1 teaspoon	5 mL
1 tablespoon	15 mL
¼ cup	59 mL
cup	79 mL
½ cup	118 mL
1 cup	177 mL

Oven Temperatures

FAHRENHEIT (F)	CELSIUS (C) (APPROXIMATE)
250°F	120 °C
300°F	150°C
325°F	165°C
350°F	180°C
375°F	190°C
400°F	200°C
425°F	220°C
450°F	230°C

Weight Equivalents

US STANDARD	METRIC (APPROXIMATE)
½ ounce	15 g
1 ounce	30 g
2 ounces	60 g
4 ounces	115 g
8 ounces	225 g
12 ounces	340 g
16 ounces or 1 pound	455 g

CPSIA information can be obtained
at www.ICGtesting.com
Printed in the USA
LVHW100819160121
676184LV00050B/495